The Tai Chi Book

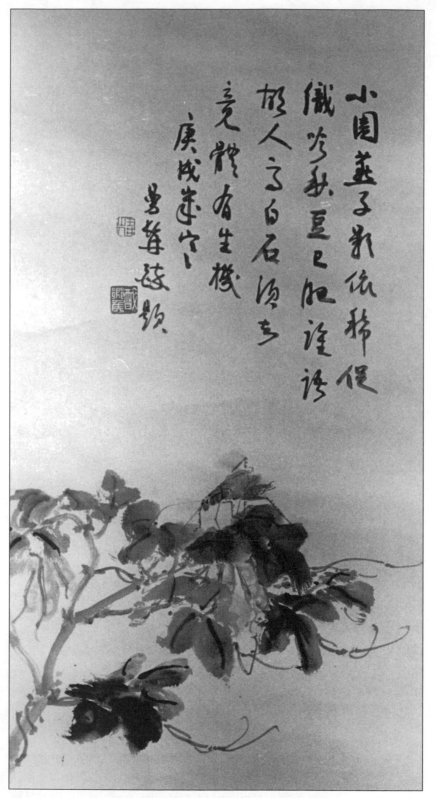

Painting by Cheng Man-ch'ing

The Tai Chi Book

Refining and Enjoying a Lifetime of Practice

Including the Teachings of Cheng Man-ch'ing,
William C. C. Chen, and Harvey I. Sober

Robert Chuckrow, Ph.D.

YMAA Publication Center
Boston, Mass. USA

YMAA Publication Center
Main Office
4354 Washington Street
Boston, Massachusetts, 02131
1-800-669-8892 • www.ymaa.com • ymaa@aol.com

10 9 8 7 6 5 4 3

ISBN:1-886969-64-7

Publisher's Cataloging in Publication
(Prepared by Quality Books Inc.)

Chuckrow, Robert.
    The tai chi book : refining and enjoying a lifetime of
practice / Robert Chuckrow ; including the teachings of Cheng
Man-ch'ing, William C. C. Chen, and Harvey I. Sober.—Rev. ed.

    p. cm. —(Martial arts—internal)
    Includes bibliographical references and index.
    ISBN 1-886969-64-7

    1. T'ai chi ch'uan. 2. Chen, William C.C.—Teachings. 3.
Cheng, Man-ch'ing—Teachings. 4. Sober, Harvey I.—Teachings.
I. Title. II. Series.

    RM727.T34C48 1998   613.7'14'8
                              QBI98-668

Cover Design by Ilana Rosenberg

Disclaimer:
The author and publisher of this material are NOT RESPONSIBLE in any manner whatsoever
for any injury which may occur through reading or following the instructions in this manual.
The activities, physical or otherwise, described in this material may be too strenuous or dangerous for some people, and the reader(s) should consult a physician before engaging in them.

Printed in Canada

Acknowledgments

I owe most of the knowledge contained herein to Cheng Man-ch'ing, William C. C. Chen, Harvey I. Sober, Don Oscar Becque, Alice Holtman, Elaine Summers, and my students, classmates, and colleagues. I am especially grateful for Stanley Israel's guidance in push-hands in recent years, which has helped me to better understand Cheng Man-ch'ing's teachings.

I thank the following people for critically reading the manuscript and making excellent suggestions: Ruth Baily, Ann Marie Baker, Dennis Capalbo, Barbara Carpenter, Philip Carter, William C. C. Chen, Helen Chuckrow, Terrence Donnely, Peggy Dillon, Barbara Drelles, Michael Ehrenreich, Moshe Eliovson, Katherine Hun Fan, Stephen Ferrari, David Franklin, Dean Gallea, Lawrence Galante, Robert Gill, Michael Gillen, Camilla Goodwyn, Neal Grossman, David Harrison, Betty Keller, Arthur Kraft, Patricia Kravit, Dr. Jeffrey Kriegel, Marian LeConte, Myles MacVane, Kathy Magee, Harley Manning, Margueritte, Judy Mayotte, Joellen McCarthy, Don Miller, Alexis Mohr, Marie Moore, Louise Parms, Madeleine Perret, Sybil Pyle, Michelle Reynolds, Roni Schweyen, Dianne Sergenian, Harvey I. Sober, Roger Staples, John Steinberg, Elaine Summers, Bryna Sweedler, Kenneth Van Sickle, Jennifer Wallace, Ed Young, Dr. Paul Yue, and Dina Zemke.

I am grateful to the following for their help with the production of the book: John Aune for answering questions about grammar and punctuation, Bill Bertche for allowing me to use his school computer at my home, Dean Gallea and Carl Ketchum for helping me transfer files, Arthur Jacobs for assisting me in the use of the Fieldston Print Shop, Lan Heng and Chung Koo Kim for patiently helping me to learn *Microsoft Word*, Carl Smith, Judy Rich, and Alex Baum-Stein for their encouragement and excellent suggestions about layout, Jinnah Hosein for helping me to scan and transfer the figures, Ruth Baily and Michael Dimeo for assisting with the photography of the postures, Kenneth Van Sickle and Robert Gill for taking some of the photographs, and Juliana Cheng for permission to use the photograph of her late husband's painting.

The one-year sabbatical granted me by the Ethical Culture Fieldston Schools, which provided time for writing this book, is gratefully acknowledged.

Contents

Author's Note x

About the Author x

Romanization of Chinese Words xi

Introduction xiii

1. What is T'ai Chi Ch'uan? 1

T'ai Chi Ch'uan as a Spiritual Teaching
T'ai Chi Ch'uan as Meditation
T'ai Chi Ch'uan as a System of Exercise, Health, and Healing
    Strength • Flexibility • Endurance • Coordination and Reflexes •
    Alignment • Knowledge of Health and Healing • Attentiveness to
    Self, Surroundings, and Nature • Patience and a Sense of Timing • Inner
    Stability and Balance • Memory • Enhanced Visualization
T'ai Chi Ch'uan as an Embodiment of Taoism
    Yin and Yang • Being in the Moment • Principle of Non-Action • The
    Concept of Zen • Non-Action in Self-Defense • Principle of Non-Intention
T'ai Chi Ch'uan as a System of Self-defense
    Some Background • How T'ai Chi Ch'uan is Used for Self-Defense
The Interconnectedness of Taoism, Health, Self-Defense, and Meditation

2. Ch'i. 18

Ch'i Kung • Some Basic Questions • What is Ch'i? • Other Benefits of Ch'i •
How is Ch'i Experienced • Is There any Scientific Basis for Ch'i? • Why
Some People Fail to Experience Ch'i • Sensing and Cultivating Ch'i • Sending
Ch'i • Effect of Clothing on Ch'i • Ch'i From Inanimate Objects • Feng Shui •
Cautions About Ch'i • To Those for Whom the Concept of Ch'i is Difficult to
Accept

3. Basic Principles and Concepts. 27

Air
Balance
    Physical Stability of Inanimate Objects • Physical Stability of People •
    How We Sense Imbalance • The Effect of Others' Actions on Balance •
    Mental Stability • Balancing of Left and Right Sides
Centering
Ch'i
Circles
Concentration
Continuity
Double Weighting
    Examples of Double Weighting
Drawing Silk
Gravity
Levelness of Motion
Leverage
Macroscopic and Microscopic Movement
Newton's First Law
Newton's Third Law
Opening and Closing of the Thigh Joints
P'eng
Perpetual Motion
    The Long River • Converting Translational Motion into Rotational Motion
Precision
Rotation

Sensitivity
    The Effect of the Mind on Sensitivity • A Physiological Factor Affecting
    Sensitivity: Weber's Law
Separation of Yin and Yang
Sequence of Motion
Shape
Spatial Relations
Stepping
    What Part of the Foot Should Contact the Ground First? • Relaxation of
    the Legs • Relaxation of the Feet • Walking Through Leaves • The
    Importance of Keeping the Center of Gravity Low During Stepping • The
    Importance of Additional Bending of the Rooted Knee During Stepping
Sticking
Strength
Sung
Suspension of the Head
Unity of Movement
Verticality of the Axis of the Body
Vision
Visualization
    Visualization in Daily life Situations

4. Breathing **58**
    Everyday Breathing
        The Importance of Efficient Breathing • Reasons for Inefficient
        Breathing • A Conjecture about the Direct Absorption of Oxygen to the
        Brain • An Abdominal Breathing Exercise
    T'ai Chi Ch'uan Breathing
        A Natural Pattern of Breathing • A Reconciliation of Different
        Breathing Patterns

5. Alignment **66**
    What is Alignment, and Why is it Important? • Why is it Necessary to Study
    Alignment? • Obstacles to Reversing Faulty Patterns • A Personal Story • A
    Story About an Acquaintance • Alignment of the Hand and Wrist • Alignment
    of the Knees • Alignment of the Ankle • Alignment of the Arch of the Foot •
    About Parallel Feet • Alignment of the Pelvis • Alignment of the Head •
    Alignment of the Shoulders • Alignment of the Elbows • Alignment of the
    Spine • Proper Sitting

6. Warm-Up and Stretching **75**
    Flexibility
        Why Do We Lose Flexibility? • Why is Flexibility Important?
    Warm-Up
    Stretching
        The Benefits of Stretching • The Importance of Stretching Correctly •
        Monitoring Progress • Arresting or Reversing Inflexibility • Experiencing
        the Effect of Each Action • Getting Up After Stretching • The Best Time
        of Day to Stretch • Yawning • Spontaneous Stretching • Stretching Using
        Gravity • Hanging • Stretching Using Momentum • The Importance of
        Stretching Equally in Both Directions • The Importance of Repeating
        Each Stretch • "Cracking" of Joints

7. Stances **83**
    Definitions of Terms
        Planes and Lines • Terms Describing Stances • Additional Terms
    Descriptions of the Main Stances
        Fifty-Fifty Stance with Straight Knees • Meditative Fifty-Fifty Stance
        • Fifty-Fifty Stance with Bent Knees • Seventy-Thirty Stance •
        Diagonal Seventy-Thirty Stance • One-Hundred-Percent Stance • A
        Note of Caution

8. On Being a Student 91

T'ai Chi Ch'uan Practice
The Importance of Practice
Class is Not Practice
Continuity of Practice
Group or Individual Practice?
How Long Should You Practice?
Indoor or Outdoor Practice?
Time of Day for Practice
Self-Discipline
Fear of Mistakes
The Mind During Practice
Ways of Practicing
At Different Speeds • Mirror Image • Blindfolded or in the Dark •
Compressed • Expanded • Extra low • On Different Surfaces • In
Different Directions or Places • In Your Mind • Stopping and
Repeating a Move or Part of a Move • Emphasizing a Principle or Idea
Supplementary Exercises
Exercises for Improving Balance
Use of a Mirror
Use of Music or a Metronome
Practice in Everyday Life
Eating Before or After Practice
"Cool-Down" of the Leg Muscles
Teachers
Choosing a Teacher
Methods of T'ai Chi Ch'uan Teachers
Asking Questions in Class
Attitude Toward the Teacher
"Perfect Masters"
Advice to Beginners
The Learning Process
Goal Orientation
A Tale about a Ruler and an Artist
How is Progress Measured?
Perfectionism
Words and Speech
Images
Critical Evaluation of Ideas
Learning From Books
Learning From a Videotape
Learning From Dreams
Taking Notes in Class
Keeping a Journal

9. Health, Healing, and Sexuality. 123

What is Health?
How is Optimal Health Attained?
Injuries
Learning from Injuries • Pain • Treating Injuries • Ch'i • Dit Da Jow •
Broken Bones Bruises • Sprains • Tendonitis • Cuts • Scrapes • Infections •
Massage • Rubs
Vision
Palming
Feet
Arches • Four Reasons Why Fallen Arches are Harmful • Rehabilitation of . . . . . .
Fallen Arches • Effect of Excessive Weight • Foot Exercises

Footwear
 Heels on Shoes • Wearing-Down of Heels • Ideal Footwear
Nutrition
 T'ai Chi Ch'uan and Optimal Body Weight
Sexuality
 Taoist Sexual Practices • Ginseng • Sex Fast
Sleep
 Naps • Sleep Amounts • Pillows

10. Miscellaneous 141

Male and Female Practitioners
Art and T'ai Chi Ch'uan
Dance and T'ai Chi Ch'uan
Science and T'ai Chi Ch'uan
Comparison of the Short and Long Forms
Variations in Interpretation of the T'ai Chi Ch'uan Movements
 Straight or Bent Rear Leg? • Why Does the Rear Foot Pivot on the
 Heel Rather Than the Toe? • Pivoting of the Empty Foot in "Brush Knee"
 • Straight or Bent Wrist? • Pre-Positioning the Rear Foot at the
 Beginning of a Movement Compared with Pivoting it at the at the End
T'ai Chi Ch'uan Compared to "Aerobic" Exercise
Other Teachings

11. Push-Hands Basics 150

One-Handed Push-Hands
Two-Handed Push-Hands
Moving Push-Hands
Basic Concepts of Push-Hands
 Concept of T'ai Chi • Yielding • Neutralization • Returning • Receiving
 Energy • Correct Force (Softness) • Rooting and Redirecting
Push-Hands Principles
 Use of Minimum Force when Neutralizing • Sticking • "Listening" •
 Non-Action • Replacement • Folding • Opposite Palms • Contacting an
 Opponent • Neutralizing Before Returning
Miscellaneous Concepts
 Importance of Stance • Circles • Equilibrium • Action and Reaction •
 Newton's Third Law and the Push-Hands Uproot • Controlling the
 Opponent's Balance • T'i Fang • Examples of T'i Fang • Mobilizing
 Intrinsic Energy • Stepping In • Grabbing • Pulling • Use of Speed •
 Push-Hands Versus Self-Defense • "Taking Punches"
Attitude
 Investment in Loss • "Feeding" the Beginner • Cooperation and Sharing
 of Knowledge Versus Competition

Appendix Postures of Cheng Man-ch'ing's Short Form 177

Names of Postures
Description of the Movements
Photographs of the Postures and Transitions

Bibliography 204

Index 206

Author's Note

Every effort has been made to be accurate and helpful. I have experienced *for myself* the truth of most of what I have put forth. However, there may be typographical errors or mistakes in content, or, some of the content may not be valid for everyone. It is my wish that the reader exercise skepticism and caution in applying the information and ideas herein—especially those in the chapter on Health, Healing, and Sexuality. The purpose of any controversial parts of this book is to stimulate the reader's thinking rather than to serve as an ultimate source of information. The book is sold with the understanding that neither the author nor publisher is engaged in rendering medical or other advice. If medical advice or other expert assistance is required, the services of a competent professional person should be sought. Therefore, neither the author nor publisher shall be held liable or responsible for any harm to anyone from the direct or indirect application of the knowledge or ideas herein.

About the Author

Robert Chuckrow has been a T'ai Chi Ch'uan practitioner since 1970 and has studied under Cheng Man-ch'ing, William C. C. Chen, and Harvey I. Sober. He has studied Structural Alignment with Don Oscar Becque, Meditation and Healing with Alice Holtman, and Kinetic Awareness with Elaine Summers. He has taught T'ai Chi Ch'uan at Shr Jung Center, Sarah Lawrence College, and in numerous community and adult-education programs. He has a Ph.D. in experimental physics, which he received from New York University in 1969 and has taught physics at New York University and The Cooper Union. He currently teaches physics at The Fieldston School in Riverdale, New York and T'ai Chi Ch'uan and Ch'i Kung in Northern Westchester, New York.

Romanization of Chinese Words

This book uses the Wade-Giles romanization system of Chinese to English. There are two other systems currently in use. These are the Pinyin and the Yale systems. The cover of this book presents the Wade-Giles romanization without apostrophies in order to simplify cataloging

Some common conversions:

Wade-Giles	Pinyin	Pronunciation
Ch'i	Qi	chē
Ch'i Kung	Qigong	chē kŭng
Ch'in Na	Qin Na	chĭn nă
Kung Fu	Gongfu	gŏng foo
T'ai Chi Ch'uan	Taijiquan	tī jē chüén

For more information, please refer to *The People's Republic of China: Administrative Atlas*, *The Reform of the Chinese Written Language*, or a contemporary manual of style.

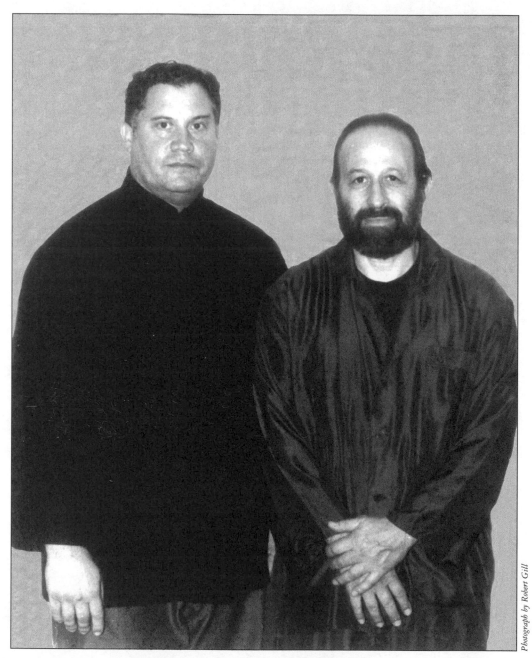

Photograph by Robert Gill

Harvey I. Sober and Robert Chuckrow

Introduction

Because of its rich heritage, T'ai Chi Ch'uan has been characterized as the pearl of Chinese culture. To the Chinese, the pearl not only has great beauty and value but also is symbolic of great wisdom. At present, T'ai Chi Ch'uan is becoming universally recognized as a high-level system of health that can benefit adults of all ages. But, in addition to health and healing, T'ai Chi Ch'uan encompasses philosophy, spirituality, and self-defense. Because it is a broad *teaching* that contains ancient wisdom and principles of action, its fascination and depth increase rather than diminish with continued study.

This book is intended to be of practical value to all who are interested in T'ai Chi Ch'uan, from the beginner to the advanced practitioner. I have striven to clarify and codify the main concepts without compromising the beauty, mystery, and tradition of T'ai Chi Ch'uan.

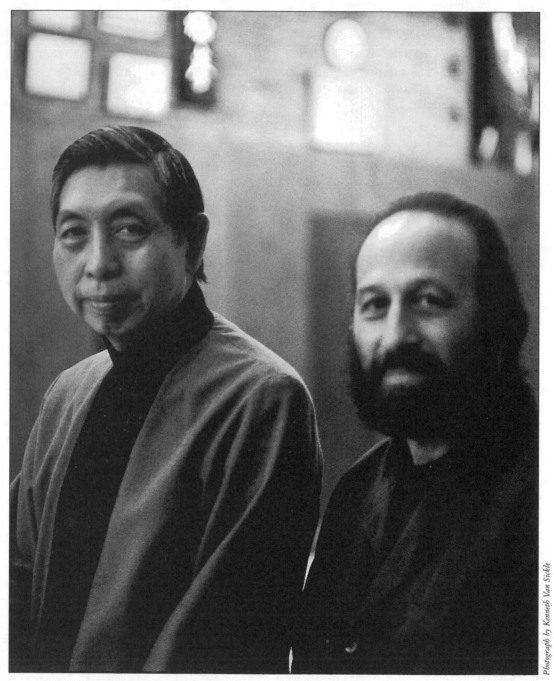

Photograph by Kenneth Van Sickle

William C. C. Chen and Robert Chuckrow

CHAPTER 1

What is T'ai Chi Ch'uan?

In April, 1970, I had been pursuing a rigorous program of calisthenics, running, and diet. I had read every book that I could on nutrition and health. An artist friend said to me, "With your interest in exercise and health, you should visit the T'ai Chi Ch'uan Association where I am studying calligraphy." With little idea of what T'ai Chi Ch'uan was, I took my friend's advice and went to Cheng Man-ch'ing's school at 211 Canal Street, in Chinatown, New York City.

Canal Street was familiar to me, as I had frequented the electronics and hardware stores there hundreds of times and eaten in numerous Chinatown restaurants. As I looked for number 211, a remarkable incident occurred. A woman whom I did not know (but who, it turned out, was a student at the school) walked up to me, pointed upward, and said, "The T'ai Chi Ch'uan school is up there."

When I walked to the inner door of the school, the first thing I noticed was a skillfully hand-lettered sign stating, "Please remove street footwear upon entering." Immediately, a tall Chinese man greeted me and invited me in to watch.

I saw a number of people dressed in a non-uniform manner, doing movements that seemed very strange to me. Many of the students did not appear to possess much physical strength. Evaluating what I saw in terms of my emphasis on muscle building, I thought to myself that these "ridiculous" movements could be of some value if they were done faster, with a ten-pound weight in each hand. As a self-righteous weight-watcher, I looked with disdain at a few students whose bodily shapes I did not associate with a school for health and fitness.

The class ended, and a different class began in which all of the students had wooden swords. A quite stocky student in this class began doing movements with impressive grace, balance, and agility. My disdain suddenly disappeared, and I reasoned that, if a person that heavy could move with such extraordinary coordination, there must be something to this strange exercise. My curiosity fully aroused, I asked the tall Chinese man what benefit I could expect from studying T'ai Chi Ch'uan. He answered, "It is different for each person." Not only did this answer intrigue me at the time, but I eventually realized the truth of it. It embodies an important Taoist precept: *Defining things limits them.*

It is impossible to convey what T'ai Chi Ch'uan is in a book of *any* length. The art must be experienced directly for a substantial period of time. The concepts of T'ai Chi Ch'uan, which have approximate parallels in physics, psychology, physiology, spiritual teachings, and religion, intertwine in a complex and mysterious manner.

Even though T'ai Chi Ch'uan is complex and is experienced uniquely by each practitioner, it is still possible to characterize it in certain respects.

T'ai Chi Ch'uan is Chinese. While no one knows exactly how old it is, it dates back, *at the very least,* to 1750 A.D. Certainly, its principles of action are rooted in knowledge and philosophy that have developed over thousands of years.

T'ai Chi Ch'uan encompasses the following five interrelated aspects. Each of these aspects will be treated in detail.

- It is a spiritual teaching.
- It is a form of meditation.
- It is a system of health and healing.
- It is the physical expression of the ancient Chinese philosophy of Taoism.
- It is a system of self-defense.

T'AI CHI CH'UAN AS A SPIRITUAL TEACHING

The main purpose in studying a spiritual teaching is to come into harmony with the universe. Many of us are out of harmony in some manner. Wars, poverty, and disease all stem from a collective lack of harmony. Addressing these problems by trying to get others to change is certainly valid. However, the basic assumption underlying most spiritual teachings is that we were placed in the world primarily for our own inner growth and, secondarily, to help others to grow. Thus, individuals must work to eliminate in *themselves* those attitudes that, on a world-wide scale, lead to war, poverty, and sickness. Through inner-growth, the individual makes a *direct* contribution to the harmony of the world but, also, influences others to change by example.

T'ai Chi Ch'uan emphasizes (a) becoming aware of the relationship of all the parts of one's body to each other and to the environment and (b) moving these parts harmoniously under the direction of the mind. For most of us, complex movement, such as walking, was learned by trial and error in a haphazard manner. Without special training, our awareness of bodily parts and their interrelationship is minimal.

Learning to move harmoniously is much more than a physical exercise. Disharmonious bodily movement is a result of faulty messages sent by the mind to the bodily parts. With practice, the student learns to send messages that result in a fluidity of movement. While the vehicle is the physical body, the development is mainly that of the mind. Practicing the movements of T'ai Chi Ch'uan strengthens bones, organs, glands, and muscles, but, at the same time, the mind is diverted from its usual mechanical mode to one that leads to increased harmony. Soon the practitioner begins to cultivate a similar harmony when approaching other pursuits.

After a student's solo movements have been sufficiently corrected, a two-person exercise called *push-hands* is taught. In push-hands practice, two students face off and alternately attack and defend using four reciprocal movements from the solo form. One main idea of push-hands is learning to yield rather than clash when attacked. Yielding does not mean that the defender gives up. In fact, T'ai Chi Ch'uan is a very effective means of defeating a skilled attacker.

Push-hands practice not only provides a foundation for self-defense but teaches principles of harmonious action. Being in harmony requires flexibility in thought and the ability to release an idea or preconception arising from the ego or societal programming. Yielding involves being in the moment instead of reacting in a routine or haphazard manner. Acting routinely (the same way every time) and acting haphazardly (in a random fashion) both involve inattentiveness. Neither of these ways of reacting takes into account the details of any particular situation. Eliminating routine or haphazard actions and replacing them by thoughtful actions predicated on centuries-old principles requires a willingness to discover and eliminate one's weaknesses. Through push-hands, practitioners become aware of their own imbalance, tension, resistance, and impulsive responses and are then able to correct them.

As students begin to see themselves clearly, there may be periods of alienation and isolation rather than connectedness to the universe as their disharmony becomes increasingly evident. Students may tend to blame themselves or others for their spiritual distress. Blaming ourselves makes taking responsibility for our actions painful. Avoidance of this pain leads to blaming others. But to blame others is to shun responsibility. This problem can be avoided by learning to observe actions without blame. Eliminating blame cultivates patience and the ability to forgive ourselves or others when we or they fall short of perfection. Push-hands practice develops a true spirit of cooperation that helps us to be objective and blameless when looking at our own or others' shortcomings. The proper practice of push-hands greatly accelerates spiritual growth and leads to true harmony.

Patience and the curbing of impulsiveness are attained through the study of T'ai Chi Ch'uan because we learn to accept our own natural rate of change. The growth process is likened to water wearing away rocks. We know from geology that water acting over sufficiently long periods of time can cause mountains to be turned into valleys. While most of us are unaware of the daily progress of geological changes, we are occasionally impressed with the cumulative effects such as rivers and gorges. Similarly, after regularly practicing the T'ai Chi Ch'uan movements over a period of time, we may suddenly become aware of how much we have changed in our approach to the world. However, this change is so natural and gradual that it is often barely noticeable.

T'AI CHI CH'UAN AS MEDITATION

Most people associate meditation with sitting in a stationary position rather than being upright and moving, as is the case with T'ai Chi Ch'uan. Let us therefore consider what meditation is in terms of the operation of the mind.

There are two main modes in which the mind operates: the mechanical and the direct. The mechanical mode is the everyday, practical one. In the mechanical mode, language is used to process sensory data from the physical world. Language is extremely powerful because it contains a body of accumulated knowledge. Unfortunately, language also contains the distortions, prejudices, opinions, and limitations of ourselves and others. Of course, the mechanical mode and its corresponding use of language has a valid function connected with our important existence in the physical world.

The direct mode is that of being in the moment. In this mode, the mind experiences directly rather than characterizing through language. The direct mode is unencumbered by self-blame, preconceptions, thoughts of either the past or future, opinions, prejudices, and limiting characterizations such as male/female, married/single, rich/poor, smart/stupid. Unfortunately, most people disregard and lose access to the direct mode.

During meditation, the mind shifts from the ordinary, mechanical mode to the direct mode for a period of time. The mind thus regains perspective by temporarily shedding the strong influences of the everyday world. In sitting meditation, the direct mode is attained by subduing the physical senses of sight, hearing, touch, smell, and taste. This shift helps to eliminate thinking in terms of language.

Activities in which the mind is keenly attuned to inner natural processes such as breathing, tension of muscles, and circulation of ch'i[1] encourage discovering and experiencing directly instead of through words. Such activities lead to a meditative state by subduing emotions, expectations, preconceptions, comparisons, and characterizations. That is why many types of meditation begin by turning the attention inward to one's breathing or to the colors and patterns "seen" through closed eyes.

T'ai Chi Ch'uan differs from sitting meditation because it involves movement and emphasizes that which enters through the senses. However, practicing T'ai Chi Ch'uan helps shift the mind from everyday cares to an attunement with inner and outer natural phenomena. Events are experienced directly rather than abstractly, through words. Therefore T'ai Chi Ch'uan is a form of meditation.

During a radio interview in his later years, J. Krishnamurti said, "Meditation is understanding one's relationship with nature and the depth of life." We think of nature as trees, birds, insects, fresh air, sunlight, clouds, etc. It is to be remembered, however, that the same laws of nature that govern trees, clouds, etc., are also manifested in each of us. T'ai Chi Ch'uan brings us into touch with nature in a direct manner. The advantage is that, with T'ai Chi Ch'uan, only a mental commitment and a four-foot by four-foot area of level floor are needed. As one of my esteemed students, Madeleine Perret, who is in her eighties, said, "T'ai Chi Ch'uan does not require much space—just a mind to do it."

> *Without leaving his door one can understand the world.*
> *Without glancing out of the window one can see the Tao of heaven.*
> *The further one travels, the less one knows.*[2]

T'ai Chi Ch'uan as a System of Exercise, Health, and Healing

For many people, exercise amounts to self-flagellation. They push and force the body beyond its limitations with little regard to the consequences. This disregard stems from goal orientation. Almost from birth, many of us are taught the erroneous idea that the result of an endeavor is more important than the process by which the result is achieved. Unfortunately, we accept this misconception.

Striving to achieve a goal by moving in a painful or harmful manner leads to an unconscious sense of vulnerability and results in a dread of exercise and even of movement itself. Stringent mental discipline is then required to initiate such exercise. Aside from causing immediate injury, forcing the body habituates faulty patterns of movement. These patterns become reflex actions, thus increasing the probability of an injury in daily life.

By contrast, if done correctly, exercise is an enjoyable, educational, and spontaneous process. Moving the body in a natural and harmonious manner gives us joy and renewed energy and generates a genuine desire to do exercise. Forms of exercise such as T'ai Chi Ch'uan teach optimal body use in daily life.

The following is a list of benefits, some of which are usually connected with exercise. These benefits are discussed in terms of the higher dimension of exercise encompassed by T'ai Chi Ch'uan.

Strength. Many people who are interested in attaining fitness overemphasize the importance of contractive muscular strength. While being strong is beneficial, it is necessary to let go of contractive muscular tension when the situation demands. The other side of strength is the ability to yield when appropriate. The entire range of *refined* (rather than *awkward*) strength, from complete relaxation to steel-like forcefulness, should be accessible to us. Instead, many untrained people are almost continually in a state of "driving with the brakes on." When one muscle is unknowingly pitted against an opposing muscle, the ability to physically react quickly and smoothly to an emergency is lost, and sensitivity to sensory stimuli is lowered. Note that muscular strength alone does not imply an ability to defend oneself. A person with a high degree of muscular strength can be easily overcome by a less muscular person who has a greater knowledge of timing and efficient body usage.

The strength of bones, organs (heart, lungs, kidneys, etc.), and the nervous system is far more important than muscular strength. In fact, health problems result more from an excess than from a deficiency of muscular strength. Fixations of muscular strength constrict organs, glands, blood vessels, and the muscles themselves. These constrictions both diminish the ability of the blood to provide nutrients and oxygen and impede the removal of wastes. Finally, muscular fixations disrupt the natural and beneficial flow of ch'i.

T'ai Chi Ch'uan strengthens the bones and vital organs. At the same time it trains the mind to send the appropriate nerve impulses to the muscles.

In T'ai Chi Ch'uan, a high degree of strength is achieved. However, this strength is not the familiar contractive strength, which is awkward and unreliable. Instead, T'ai Chi Ch'uan cultivates relaxed but expansive strength. More will be said on the distinction between contractive and expansive strength in chapter 3.

Flexibility. Flexibility has two aspects: extensibility and pliability.

Extensibility is the ability of the muscles to move through the full range allowed by the physiological structure of the joints. We are born with a full range of extensibility. This range diminishes because of misuse or lack of use of our bodies. With educated use, such deterioration need not occur and can actually be reversed.

Pliability is the ability to adapt to the situation at hand through movement and requires that the mind send appropriate messages to the muscles to use whatever range of extensibility the person possesses. It is possible for a person to be potentially quite flexible but not be flexible when it is required. This deficiency results from the improper processing of sensory data and from a consequent lack of appropriate nerve impulses to the muscles. T'ai Chi Ch'uan trains us to process sensory data and react quickly, efficiently, and appropriately in an unexpected situation. Thus, the meditative, self-defense, and health aspects merge.

Endurance. We tend to think of endurance in the context of temporarily demanding activities such as a race or the repeated lifting of a weight. Another facet of endurance, however, is that of persevering over an extended period of time, patiently using knowledge of natural rates rather than trying to accomplish things all at once. The concept of endurance is an important aspect of Kung Fu.[3] True perseverance also involves knowing when to stop, when to rest, and when to turn to another activity in order to optimize progress over the long haul.

Here, goal orientation plays a significant role. It is common for those who are pursuing what would otherwise be a constructive regimen, to overdo, thereby squandering their effort. In some cases severe harm is done by pushing the body beyond its limits. It is not hard to find cases of athletes who have suffered injuries this way. Sometimes it takes more self-discipline to limit one's activity than to overdo it. It requires an inner security to know that, with perseverance over time, a beneficial result will inevitably occur.

Coordination and Reflexes. *Coordination* is the ability of the mind to direct the body parts to move efficiently and harmoniously. *Reflexes* are spontaneous responses to situations and occur without conscious thought. Properly coordinated reflex actions result from prior repetition of similar coordinated actions. Coordination is developed by doing movements slowly and meditatively so that the mind can process them. Reflexes are the result of sufficient repetition to form well trodden neural pathways. Because the practice of T'ai Chi Ch'uan requires a continuous mental involvement in all movements, the receiving, processing, and sending of neural impulses is developed to a high degree.

Alignment. In many physical pursuits other than T'ai Chi Ch'uan, the alignment of the body parts is learned by trial and error. Even such a basic skill as walking is learned in this manner. Such a haphazard process of development often results in habitual faulty alignment of bones.

Faulty alignment can result in damaging stress on joints. Knees and ankles are especially vulnerable because they bear the weight of the body. These joints are far more susceptible to being sprained when poorly aligned.

Chronic stress of joints can cause cartilage to wear away, precipitating arthritis. With years of misuse, affected joints manifest the literal grinding of bone against bone rather than the frictionless gliding action of the smooth, lubricated cushion provided by healthy cartilage.

It is important that the physiologically correct alignment of body parts be learned and habituated as early as possible. The chance of a joint injury is greatly reduced once proper alignment is achieved. I have seen practitioners (including myself) quickly recover from long-term knee problems after correcting faulty alignment.

Alignment is also related to overall strength. When the bones line up properly, less muscular strength is required to achieve a given result.

Because the movements of T'ai Chi Ch'uan are slow and meditative, they provide an ideal vehicle for the study and improvement of alignment. Alignment is discussed in detail in chapter 5.

Knowledge of Health and Healing. Most people do not take responsibility for their own health. Martial artists (and T'ai Chi Ch'uan practitioners in particular) become so highly attuned to every facet of the body's functioning that when something is wrong, they promptly detect it. They are then able to direct the life force or arrange conditions to facilitate the reversal of bodily injury at an early stage, before the damage becomes a serious medical problem. Some routinely treat bruises, pulled muscles, sprains, and minor burns effectively on their own.

The following story will help to illustrate the degree of self-sufficiency of some practitioners of martial arts: When I was studying Aikido for a while under Marilyn Fountain, she came to class one day with a broken index finger. This injury had occurred while practicing with a classmate of hers the day before. To demonstrate to us that the finger was broken, she wiggled it midway between two successive joints. She said that she had been unsuccessfully trying to set the finger herself. When she came to class the following week, her finger was the same. However, the week after that, she had finally managed to set the bone and showed that she could move her finger in a completely normal manner. She said, "During the second week, the break started to become sticky, and with a little experimentation it was easy to feel when the bones fit together perfectly." She had set the bone without X-rays or splints—and without medical intervention.

Here is another story: While visiting a friend in the country, I was carving something with a pen knife. The knife slipped and caused a very deep gash across the palm of my hand near the base of my thumb. My friend became quite upset and pleaded with me to go to a hospital. I insisted on taking care of the matter myself. I closed the wound by taping my thumb to my little finger with clear surgical tape. Next, I cleaned the surface of the wound with moist cotton, mated the edges as perfectly as possible, and covered it with surgical tape. After a few days, the wound had healed sufficiently to remove the tape safely. After about a week, a little trace of the wound was visible, although the inside was not yet completely healed. It took about a month for the wound to heal to the degree that there was no pain whatsoever under normal use. Today there is only the faintest trace of a very thin scar that has to be carefully pointed out for another person to notice it. The natural lines on my skin that traverse the scar match perfectly even when viewed with a magnifying glass. The skin and underlying flesh are now soft, pliable, and normal in every respect.

It is to be emphasized that the preceding two stories are included for the purpose of illustrating a degree of self-sufficiency that it is possible to gradually develop through many years of study. Self-remedy of this sort is certainly not recommended to the reader.

Another facet of T'ai Chi Ch'uan is the incorporation of self-massage. Massage is commonly thought of only in terms of muscles. Nevertheless, the skin, bones, organs, glands, blood vessels, and nerves all benefit from massage.

Massage improves the circulation of blood, lymph, and ch'i (see chapter 2 for a discussion of ch'i) to the region involved. This combined circulation helps to wash away toxins and bring the nutrients required for healing. Massage sensitizes the area involved and aids in the early discovery of problems that, otherwise, might go unnoticed and make treatment excessively lengthy or even impossible. The resulting sensitization also has an educational effect of an increased awareness of how muscles, etc., are used. This awareness conduces to improved usage, alignment, and relaxation.

Massage will be discussed in more detail in chapter 9.

Attentiveness to Self, Surroundings, and Nature. Unlike many other exercises, T'ai Chi Ch'uan improves the connection between body and mind; we become aware of our habitual patterns of movement and our impulses of action. Those who practice T'ai Chi Ch'uan movements relate their body parts to each other, the ground, and gravity. The awareness of these elements is an important benefit. Push-hands practice builds a particular awareness of the motives of others and of one's range of effect on others.

A philosophical concept central to T'ai Chi Ch'uan that is discussed later in this chapter is *being in the moment*. This concept means concentrating and focusing the attention in the here and now rather than allowing the attention to be diverted or scattered. We thereby increase our powers of observation and, thus, our ability to learn.

Attentiveness to nature has already been discussed. Those out of touch with nature become caught in a vicious cycle that makes them unable to relate their consequent disharmony to anything meaningful to themselves. Thus, they are prone to anxiety, depression, and ill health and lack the ability to correct these disorders.

Patience and a Sense of Timing. Impulsiveness stems from a lack of both patience and proper timing. Patience and timing require an awareness of the natural rates of processes and a willingness not to force a result to occur prematurely. To this end, the T'ai Chi Ch'uan practitioner learns not to overdo or underdo. Moderation is essential in any exercise if progress is to be maximized and injury minimized.

Inner Stability and Balance. Improved physical balance is a benefit of correct exercise. Mental balance is a more difficult achievement.

The practice of T'ai Chi Ch'uan releases undesirable muscular tensions, resulting in physical improvements. These tensions ultimately stem from the manner in which the mind governs the body. The release of such tensions can result only from a release of corresponding mental fixations. Therefore, practice of T'ai Chi Ch'uan slowly cultivates a mind that is increasingly able to change when needed. True mental stability occurs when the mind adjusts and releases instead of rigidly adhering to an idea.

Another benefit is that T'ai Chi Ch'uan uses the whole body on both sides, thereby balancing the opposite sides of the brain. Balanced usage will be discussed in detail in chapter 3.

Memory. According to memory experts, a major cause of poor memory is inattentiveness. Memory improves when proper attentiveness is achieved. In T'ai Chi Ch'uan and other disciplines of depth, the memory is challenged by a large number of concepts and intricate movements. Because the practitioner is highly attentive during class and practice, memory for movement improves noticeably.

When I started studying T'ai Chi Ch'uan, I had such difficulty in remembering new movements that, in each weekly class, I hoped that a new movement would not be taught. Unfortunately, I found that I could not do any but the beginning movements at home. After being a student for a few years, my memory for movement had improved so much that my classmate under Cheng Man-ch'ing, friend, and colleague, Lawrence Galante, was able to teach me the entire T'ai Chi Broadsword form in just four fifty-minute lessons.

Enhanced Visualization. When exercise is sufficiently complex to actively engage the mind, the powers of visualization are challenged and thereby improved. The T'ai Chi Ch'uan form and push-hands are very difficult to master. On all levels of ability it is necessary that the mind coordinate the movement of all of the parts of the body in relation to each other and in relation to the movements of others. This coordination requires an active process of visualization.

T'AI CHI CH'UAN AS AN EMBODIMENT OF TAOISM

The above eleven benefits are all closely interrelated through Taoist philosophical principles. According to Taoist (pronounced *dau'ist*) philosophy, all qualities span a range of complementary pairs, called *yin* and *yang*. The Taoist concept of continually balancing yin and yang is called *T'ai Chi* (literally, *supreme ultimate*). Since Ch'uan means fist, *T'ai Chi Ch'uan* is a system of self-defense based on the balancing of yin and yang. That is why *T'ai Chi Ch'uan* is sometimes called *Taoist Boxing*.

Yin and Yang. Examples of complementary pairs of some familiar qualities are given in Table 1-1. The reader might also examine the synopsis of categories at the beginning of a Roget's Thesaurus,[4] which organizes complementary aspects of every imaginable quality. Then determine which aspect is yin and which is yang.

Quality	Yin	Yang
gender	female	male
pressure	soft	hard
temperature	cold	hot
visible light	reflected	radiated
force	weak	strong
sensation	insubstantial	substantial
taste	sweet	salty
capacity	empty	full
concept	intangible	tangible
action	yielding	standing firm
learning	passive	active
	absorbing	expressing
	observing	doing
direction	down (earth)	up (heaven/ch'i)
	left	right
	backward	forward

Table 1-1. *The yin and yang aspects of some familiar qualities.*

Viewing things in terms of yin and yang might seem to be a gross oversimplification. In fact, it is not. The Westerner is highly accustomed to precision and may fail to realize that these categories are only the *surface* of a profound conceptual framework. The concept of T'ai Chi seems simple but, in actuality, takes much time to comprehend.

There is a yin-yang range of each action we take in any situation. Each action must have the right proportion of yin and yang to be in harmony with nature. An understanding of yin and yang helps us to put these aspects in balance. This balance is represented by the T'ai Chi symbol (see Fig. 1-1).

Since the black part of the T'ai Chi symbol is the presence of something tangible, namely ink, it might seem that it should be yang. Similarly, the white part is the absence of anything and would be yin. However, this perspective is incorrect. As abstract entities, white and black symbolize light and darkness, respectively. Light is substantial and darkness is insubstantial. Thus, the white part represents yang and the black part represents yin.

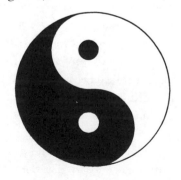

Fig. 1-1. *The T'ai Chi symbol. The dark part is yin, and the light part is yang.*

Note that the T'ai Chi symbol portrays yin and yang as continuously evolving from one to another, as night into day. When yang becomes full, it starts to become yin, and vice versa. If an action is too strong, it will produce weakness. Conversely, yielding to a strong attack results in a stronger position. Moreover, since nothing is completely yin or completely yang, the fullest yin part contains a small circular region of yang, and vice versa.

> *Nothing in the world is softer and more supple than water,*
> *Yet when attacking the hard and the strong, nothing can surpass it.*
> *The supple overcomes the hard.*
> *The soft overcomes the strong.*
>
> —Lao Tzu, (Ch. 78)

Note that neither yin nor yang can be characterized as good or bad. We tend to think of standing firm as good and yielding as bad. This misconception results from a lack of harmony with nature and from taking a simple-minded approach. Nature is neutral, and its range cannot be simplified in terms of good and bad.

Let us examine life and death in terms of yin and yang. We think of life as being good and death as bad. How could these be considered to be complementary and neutral?

Asian philosophies and religions, early Christianity, and even Judaism[5] accept the concept of reincarnation. Viewed in the light of reincarnation, death is more than dying. In this view, death is one's state after life and commences with the act of dying. A more balanced characterization would be *life* and *afterlife*. Life and afterlife can be thought of as evolving one into the other and as part of a reciprocal process, neither counterpart of which can be considered as good or bad.

While no one should accept reincarnation on the authority of others, keeping an open mind is of prime importance in dealing with new ideas. An open mind allows a proper balance between the ideas of others and one's own direct experience.

Being in the Moment. Being in the moment does not imply being recklessly self indulgent or oblivious to the past or future. On the contrary, it implies coordinating past, present, and future. Being in the moment requires using concentration and creative faculties to intensify the effectiveness of any action. The idea is to confront any need for correction or adaptation to a continually changing environment rather than letting things slide, with gaps in attentiveness.

> *Plan to tackle the difficult when it is easy.*
> *Undertake the great when it is small.*
> *Begin the most difficult task in the world when it is still easy.*
> *Begin the greatest task in the world when it is still small.*
> *That is how the Sage becomes great without striving.*
>
> —Lao Tzu, (Ch. 63)

In every moment of each of our lives, circumstances require us to react in some manner, either for our own self-preservation or for the manifestation of our purpose in the universe. Living structures consisting of single cells can react to their environment only through direct physical means. By contrast, human beings possess highly complex organs that sense and process goings-on in the world long before these impinge directly. We fall short of living up to our full potential to the extent that there are lapses in this sensing and processing.

T'ai Chi Ch'uan practice cultivates an expanded awareness of the movement of all body parts in relation to each other and to gravity, in accordance with a set of underlying principles. One such principle, which will be discussed in detail in chapter 3, is "centering." Joints are *centered* when they are in a neutral alignment rather than towards an extreme. As one moves, the effect of gravity, which pulls joints away from center, constantly changes. Thus, continual minute adjustments of inner tension are required to keep the joints centered.

The beginner tends either to apply gross tension or to have large gaps in concentration, resulting in sudden spastic readjustments. As the connection between mind and body becomes more continuous, the movements display a corresponding continuity. Here, continuity is an outward manifestation of *being in the moment.*

An important dividend of being in the moment during practice is that the mind becomes increasingly capable of involvement in any action, not just that which is practiced. Of course, the rate of improvement of what is practiced is maximized, with corresponding benefits such as improved balance and coordination, circulation of blood and ch'i to organs, the releasing of muscular tension, the subduing of mechanical thinking, and decreased vulnerability to injury in everyday movements. Additionally, one may notice a greater focus in other activities such as sports, playing a musical instrument, writing, driving a car, etc.

The increased efficiency of being focused and being in the moment results in minimal outer action, a concept that is discussed next.

Principle of Non-Action. Blaise Pascal (1623-1662), ended a long letter with the apologetic remark, "I have made this letter rather long only because I have not had the time to make it shorter."[6] Often, doing less is not easy. However, cultivating improved efficiency on a daily basis results in less and less action, the logical limit of which is "*non*-action."

One of the basic concepts in T'ai Chi Ch'uan is to *neither overdo nor underdo.* (In most actions we tend to overdo.) A saying involving this concept is, "In T'ai Chi Ch'uan the hands do not move." This saying sounds paradoxical. In order to glean the hidden meaning we must first note that this statement contradicts the obvious: The hands *do* move.

Such statements shun the kind of scientific precision to which we Westerners are accustomed. Rather, by repudiating the obvious, they illuminate a higher meaning: Moving the hands by using contractive muscular action is to be eliminated. Scientifically speaking, the hands move in space, but their motion *relative to the body* is minor.

In order for the hands to move with the minimum of contractive strength, the practitioner must uncover inefficiencies, tensions, impulsiveness, etc., and strip these away. The problem is that we are so familiar with these unnecessary tensions that they do not subside without a major effort. Herein lies an apparent paradox: in order to move efficiently without thought, one must engage in intense concentration for a period of time.

The Concept of Zen. Although Zen is associated with Japanese philosophy, it originated in China and then spread to Japan. Chan, as it was called in China, can be thought of as the marriage of Buddhism and Taoism.

The Zen concept of correct action without thought or volition is attained only through the application of both action and volition during the initial stages of learning. Action and volition must precede effective non-action. The Zen masters had previously achieved high proficiency in a discipline by conventional means. The practice of Zen was a means of transcending the eventual limitations of conventional practice. Acting "without thought" is meaningful only after one has methodically and deliberately built a strong foundation.

My first teacher, Cheng Man-ch'ing, could create beautiful paintings and works of calligraphy effortlessly in minutes. Nevertheless, he required his beginning students of calligraphy and painting to draw hundreds of straight lines every day for months. I remember seeing these students assiduously painting closely spaced lines on full sheets of newspaper. First, they drew horizontal lines in alternating directions. Then vertical lines were likewise drawn. When a sheet finally looked like graph paper, they discarded it and repeated the process on a fresh sheet.

The creative dimension emerges only after the initial stage of learning is mastered. Then Zen begins.

> *One who thinks everything is easy inevitably finds everything difficult.*
> *That is why the Sage alone regards everything as difficult and in the end*
> *finds no difficulty at all.*
> —Lao Tzu (Ch. 63)

A similar thought is expressed in the following:

> *My method is to take the utmost trouble to find the right thing to say, and*
> *then to say it with the utmost levity.*[7]
> —George Bernard Shaw

Non-Action in Self-Defense. All wasteful action is considered to be a cardinal sin in self-defense. Any wasteful action in a critical situation puts the practitioner at a disadvantage because valuable time is lost. Moreover, wasteful actions "telegraph" intention to the opponent, who can use this against the practitioner.

Principle of Non-Intention. Sigmund Freud, the father of modern psychoanalysis, originated the term *free-floating attention*. By this term, Freud meant that, to understand a situation, one must let go of all preconceptions and be empty, thereby allowing creative insight to penetrate.

> *In pursuing knowledge, one accumulates daily.*
> *In practicing Tao, one loses daily.*
>
> —Lao Tzu, (Ch. 48)

In the practice of the T'ai Chi Ch'uan solo form, we shed any prior ideas of how a body should move. Observing the natural manner in which all body parts move develops an open and efficient approach to learning. Similarly, in push-hands practice, we follow the moves of our partner rather than coercing him/her into a weaker position. Professor Cheng termed this approach *investment in loss.* At the beginning, false results can be obtained by incorrect means, e.g., using contractive muscular strength. Cultivation of the correct principles means foregoing initial false success but makes one stronger in the long run.

T'AI CHI CH'UAN AS A SYSTEM OF SELF-DEFENSE

Some Background. Because T'ai Chi Ch'uan is so peaceful, it is possible for some who study T'ai Chi Ch'uan never to think of it as pertaining to fighting. Nevertheless, T'ai Chi Ch'uan is a martial art. In fact, at one time T'ai Chi Ch'uan was the most highly regarded system of fighting and was kept a strict secret by the members of the Chen family. About a century-and-a-half ago, Yang Lu-Chan was a servant for the Chen family. Legend has it that one night Yang awoke before dawn. Hearing a commotion in the courtyard, he investigated and saw the Chen family secretly practicing T'ai Chi Ch'uan. Yang recognized the high level of training he witnessed. Thereafter, he watched night after night.

One night during practice, there was an occurrence that was so exciting that Yang forgot himself and yelled out. He was discovered and was then required to show what he knew. Because he had absorbed so much of what he had seen, Yang was "adopted" by the Chen family and was taught T'ai Chi Ch'uan freely.

Yang went on to become a famous fighter and win many tournaments. As a result, he was summoned to teach the Imperial Court T'ai Chi Ch'uan. Because he could not reveal what he had been secretly taught, he originated a modified version that would also be more suitable to aristocrats for whom it would be inappropriate to do certain highly martial movements. Nevertheless, Yang retained the essential philosophical concepts. "Yang-style" T'ai Chi Ch'uan then became public.

Today the Chen style is still secret, although modified public versions exist. The Chen style remains the most martial and retains explosive and physically demanding movements interspersed with subtle ones. The Yang style is more subdued. While the Yang style is a powerful system of fighting, many Yang-style practitioners pursue the health and spiritual aspects more than the martial aspects.

My first teacher, Cheng Man-ch'ing, studied with Yang Cheng-fu, a grandson of Yang Lu-chan. Cheng introduced a number of modifications, the most notable of which is a short version of the solo form (outlined in the Appendix). Other short versions have since emerged.

How T'ai Chi Ch'uan is Used for Self-Defense. T'ai Chi Ch'uan is in sharp contrast to other martial arts that utilize blocking techniques requiring strength and speed. Instead of meeting an incoming attack with force, the T'ai Chi Ch'uan practitioner permits only a very light contact. The attacker expects a forceful resistance whether the attack succeeds or is blocked and exerts corresponding forces against the ground in order to maintain balance against the expected resistance of the opponent. The absence of the expected resistance "neutralizes" the attack and causes the attacker to become momentarily unbalanced and overextended. It is said, "From the sentence *A force of four ounces deflects a thousand pounds* we know that the technique is not accomplished with strength."[8] The T'ai Chi Ch'uan practitioner then "seizes the moment before the attacker has a chance to recover from an inferior position."

In order to achieve a level where such neutralization can reliably occur, it is necessary to practice for a much longer period of time than is needed to achieve a corresponding martial skill in other arts such as Karate. Therefore, many regard the health, spiritual, and philosophical aspects as the main reason for studying T'ai Chi Ch'uan.

Even though the self-defense aspect is not always emphasized, it should not be disregarded because it ensures that the integrity of the principles is maintained. Self-defense practice ideally incorporates the basic T'ai Chi Ch'uan philosophy of cooperation and harmony.

THE INTERCONNECTEDNESS OF TAOISM, HEALTH, SELF-DEFENSE, AND MEDITATION

Thousands of years ago in China, there were people who wanted to find the way to immortality. At that time, to be free, people had to be able to defend their lives at a moment's notice. Those without fighting skills were easy prey to others who would enslave and exploit them. Once enslaved, a person would be so drained of life force that pursuing the way to immortality would be out of the question.

Only those who were proficient in martial arts could freely pursue cultural and spiritual activities such as music, art, calligraphy, and philosophy. Some of these martial artists realized that the reason for ill health and spiritual distress was a lack of inner harmony. The mortality of the human body was attributed to the concept that the mind, which dictates how the body will act, is incognizant of the true nature of the body and the world. Thus it was thought that the mind got the body into trouble through wrong thinking.

The Chinese have always been highly attuned to nature. To this day, young Chinese children are taught about the insects, animals, and sounds of nature. Thousands of years ago, people lived in even closer contact with nature than is the case today. Thus it was felt that the study of nature and the consequent application of nature's principles to human endeavors would lead to the attainment of immortality and right action. The human body was regarded as an object of nature similar to clouds, water, air, and the different animals. The goal was for the mind, which governs and dwells in the body, to come into harmony with the laws of nature. Attaining this goal required emptying the mind of its preconceptions, distortions, and wasteful preprogrammed responses. The mind would then be able to allow the body to act in a natural and efficient manner. Only after the mind was in harmony with both the body and the life-force of nature could immortality be attained.

> *Who can still the muddy water and gradually make it clear?*
> *Who can make the still gradually become alive through activity?*
> *Just because they are not full they can avoid wearing out and*
> *being replaced.*
>
> —Lao Tzu, (Ch. 15)

Those who espoused this Taoist philosophy believed that it applied to every endeavor, including self-defense. The same laws of nature that pertain to longevity also provide protection from the deadly attack of a trained person. The most stringent test of whether a philosophy of action is legitimate is if it can be used for self-defense. If you are able to withstand the attack of someone who is trained to see and utilize your weaknesses, then you are correspondingly less vulnerable to random pitfalls of a less insidious nature. Thus, the Taoist principles of health became interwoven with fighting. Fighting gestures and movements merged with those used to cultivate the life force.

Spiritual teachings hold that the purpose of life is to come into harmony with universal laws. These laws are manifested in nature. Therefore, a system that leads to attunement with nature is a spiritual teaching.

It can be seen that the philosophical, spiritual, health, and self-defense aspects of T'ai Chi Ch'uan are beautifully interconnected.

Notes

1. The concept of ch'i is of such importance that the next chapter is entirely devoted to its discussion.

2. Lao Tzu: "My words are easy to understand," *Lectures on the Tao Teh Ching by Man-jan Cheng,* Translated by Tam C. Gibbs, North Atlantic Books, 1981, Ch. 47.

3. While many associate the term Kung Fu solely with martial arts, it refers to the achievement of skill in any endeavor by means of leisurely persistence over a substantial period of time.

4. Peter Mark Roget, *Roget's International Thesaurus,* Harper Collins Publishers, New York, NY, 1992, pp. xix–xxv.

5. See Gershom Scholem, *Kabbalah,* Keter Publishing House, Jerusalem, 1974, pp. 344–350.

6. Blaise Pascal, *Lettres Provinciales,* 14 Dec, 1656.

7. George Bernard Shaw, *Answers to Nine Questions.*

8. From Wang Tsung-yueh's *T'ai-Chi Ch'uan Lun.* See *The Essence of T'ai-Chi Ch'uan: The Literary Tradition,* Edited by Benjamin Pang-jeng Lo et al., North Atlantic Books, Berkeley, CA, 1985, p. 37.

CHAPTER 2

Ch'i

Ch'i is unlimited. Take as much as you like—
no one will ever accuse you of being greedy.

—Cheng Man-ch'ing

Correct practice of T'ai Chi Ch'uan includes the cultivation of a highly valued entity called *Ch'i.*[1] *Ch'i* is a Chinese term corresponding to no word in English; in fact, no Western concept is even remotely related to it. The Japanese call it *ki,* and in India it is called *prana.* Some translators use the words breath, blood, energy, or life force in describing ch'i. While blood and oxygen are important accompaniments to ch'i, these characterizations are quite insufficient.

Ch'i Kung

In China and neighboring countries, the existence of ch'i is widely accepted. Many Chinese devote a substantial portion of their time to a discipline called Ch'i Kung (pronounced chee gung). Ch'i Kung is the skill of concentrating, circulating, and focusing ch'i. In China, multitudes of people practice Ch'i Kung every morning in the parks. There are magazines and books dedicated to Ch'i Kung. Traditional Chinese medicine takes ch'i into account. Even the design of buildings is based on considerations of ch'i.

Ch'i Kung practitioners experience the ch'i to flow along paths in the body called meridians. Acupuncture is based on a knowledge of ch'i and its meridians. At its highest level, acupuncture involves injecting ch'i at just the right time and place and in the right amount to reinstate its natural flow in the patient.

Ch'i embodies antithetical qualities: it can be used for healing, or it can be used for breaking stones (or bones). Only the healing aspect of ch'i will be discussed in this book.

Some Basic Questions

How can it be that many people in one part of the world acknowledge the existence of ch'i and even base their system of medicine on it, while those in other parts of the world have no concept of it? What is ch'i? How is it experienced? How is it cultivated? Can it be sent from one person to another? Do inanimate objects have ch'i? Does ch'i have any scientific basis? Does it need such a basis? These questions will be addressed next.

What is Ch'i?

We think of the physical human body as being composed of bones, muscles, tendons, ligaments, organs, glands, nerves, blood, lymph, etc. However, there is one more component in living human bodies: ch'i. Ch'i is regarded as that which regulates the functioning and mutual interaction of all the bodily organs. When we are physically injured, the obvious damage is accompanied by a disruption of the flow of ch'i. One of the causes of this interruption is our pain and fear. If the flow of ch'i is not reinstated, the recovery process is hampered or even absent.

Ch'i Kung and T'ai Chi Ch'uan practitioners are sensitive to the flow of ch'i and can reinstate its flow. The time required for healing seems to be proportional to the length of time that the flow of ch'i has been disrupted. If a strong flow of ch'i is reinstated immediately after an injury, the healing process will be very short—perhaps only a few days. Frequently, pain subsides in minutes. However, if a period of time elapses before the ch'i is reinstated, the healing process may be markedly delayed. Consequently, there are certain types of injuries (such as bruises, sprains, muscle spasms, and burns) that have a potential for a much shorter recovery time than is commonly thought.

Other Benefits of Ch'i

In addition to hastening recovery from injury and illness, regular practice of Ch'i Kung promotes a feeling of dynamo-like energy, lessens the need for sleep, reduces the tendency to become sick, and makes the whole body physically resilient and strong.

It should be noted that, often, beginners first feel tired rather than energized when they practice T'ai Chi Ch'uan or Ch'i Kung. This disappointing effect is actually good because it is important to become aware of the body's needs. The tiredness occurs mainly because most people consume fatigue-masking stimulants such as caffeine or "hypnotize" themselves not to experience their fatigue. Once those with an energy deficit relax, they realize how tired they are.

The body becomes inefficient when we postpone the opportunity for it to perform metabolic cleansing, nutritive functions, and the balancing of the actions of the various organs. Thus, the energy debt keeps escalating. Ch'i Kung practice gives the whole body a chance to undergo the beneficial transformations before harm mounts. Bodily and mental energy then gradually increase rather than decline with time.

In the words of one of my Chinese students at Fieldston School, "My father says that if he did not wake up every morning at five o'clock and do an hour of Ch'i Kung, he would not be able to work fourteen hours a day."

How is Ch'i Experienced?

The most common description of ch'i is a tingling or squirming sensation. This sensation is often mistaken by beginners to be that of the circulation of the blood, but the movement of blood causes more of a pulsing feeling.

As the practitioner becomes more adept, a swelling sensation begins to appear. The swelling has a supportive quality that pervades the entire body without any gaps and makes it possible to exert surprisingly large amounts of external force in a totally relaxed and natural manner.

Advanced practitioners experience ch'i *circulating* through the body. The circulation of ch'i is enhanced by movement or by mental intent.

Is There Any Scientific Basis for Ch'i?

While some research has been conducted, scientists have not yet satisfactorily identified, measured, or explained ch'i. Therefore, it is misleading to try to describe ch'i using words like *energy* or *force*. Such words have precise scientific meanings that may not apply. However, ch'i is not altogether without scientific basis. Here is a biological interpretation of ch'i, based on ideas taught to me by Elaine Summers, with whom I studied "Kinetic Awareness" in New York City in the mid 1970's:

When we look at dead cells under a microscope, they are motionless. We know about their changes by seeing them "frozen" at different stages of development. However, there is a dynamic attribute of living cells similar to that seen in living, single-celled organisms such as amoebas. Living cells undergo a movement that is termed *protoplasmic streaming*. Streaming allows oxygen, nutrients, and metabolic wastes to pass in their appropriate directions through the cell wall. In tissues comprising many cells, there may be a similar activity involving masses of cells in unison—a sort of wave-like undulation. The effect of a combined, intelligent, unified motion may well transmit vital information from each organ and gland to every other organ and gland. This explanation is consistent with the concept that ch'i, blood, and breath are related and that ch'i harmonizes the essential bodily functions. It is also consistent with the fact that ch'i is often experienced as a tingling sensation and its flow is experienced as a wave.

The idea that ch'i involves such vital cellular activities explains why its presence is associated with a healing effect. When protoplasmic streaming is arrested, it stunts normal physiological processes dependent on this streaming. Reinstated normal streaming then causes those physiological processes to resume. If this interpretation is correct, then exercises that cultivate the flow of ch'i benefit cells individually as well as allowing them to harmonize collectively.

At present, some people who work with ch'i say that it involves electromagnetic energy. Electronic devices have been designed that are purported to sense ch'i. These devices are used by some acupuncturists to locate the acupuncture nodes. While ch'i may well involve electromagnetic energy, this involvement is certainly not the whole answer. When it comes to pursuits of self-cultivation, we must be careful that scientific clarity and efficiency do not limit that which is ideally experienced directly.

Why Some People Fail to Experience Ch'i

Ch'i is a subtle phenomenon that occurs in all of us. If your ch'i stopped, you would cease to be alive. If ch'i is such a natural part of life, why is it that many people do not feel it without some sort of training? One explanation is that, because we experience ch'i from the very inception of our lives, we become so used to it that it goes unnoticed. This disregard is true of other familiar natural processes such as the flow of blood throughout our body, changes in concentration of oxygen of the blood from breath to breath, the flow of digestive juices, the absorption of nutrients after they are digested, and the emptying of the stomach. As long as these processes are not under stress, we are usually not aware of them. However, those who study teachings such as Yoga or T'ai Chi Ch'uan become highly attuned to all of these processes and more.

There is another reason that awareness of biological activities is often faint. Such an awareness saps energy from practical tasks. If we were consciously aware of every beat of our heart, every movement of our digestive tract, and other processes, we would be so distracted that we would be aware of little else. Fortunately, the mind has the ability to cut off its awareness of certain things almost totally. For example, while you are reading this page, there are many stimuli that do not enter into your awareness. There is the pressure of the chair against the back of your thighs (if you are sitting), there may be sounds of automotive traffic, airplanes, animals, insects, music, and speech. In order to concentrate on what is of immediate importance, it is necessary to suspend the processing of extraneous stimuli. Often we do this so well that even important sensory input is obliterated.

Each of us has been exposed to our own internal circulation of blood since shortly after the egg from which we grew was fertilized. However, the fact that the blood circulates was discovered by Western medicine only a few hundred years ago. Therefore, it should not be surprising that without special training, many people do not experience the similarly subtle flow of ch'i.

Sensing and Cultivating Ch'i

Probably the most important precondition for the serious cultivation of ch'i is a state called sung. Sung is discussed in detail in chapter 3, but, for the present discussion, it will suffice to describe sung as a state of inner relaxation without any compromise of outer shape. Once a certain degree of sung is attained, it is then helpful to notice the circulation of the blood and its oxygenation. Another help is to feel the flow of air over the skin during slow movement. This feeling is somewhat similar to that of ch'i. A third help is to gently "squeeze" and "stretch" the space between the fingers. This squeezing can also be applied to the space between the hands and to the space between the arms and the body. Achieving the correct degree of tension and openness will result in a distinct energizing and tingling of the parts involved.

After one's movements are sufficiently relaxed and fluid, it is important to notice subtle changes of internal pressure that occur with every movement. The practitioner will then begin to sense a *flow* of ch'i. Eventually, awareness of the familiar route that the ch'i takes will become strong. This awareness is then used to make minute changes in the speed, tension, and shape of the movements to increase the strength of the natural flow of ch'i. Developing this awareness is called *cultivating the ch'i*.

In the T'ai Chi Ch'uan form, the mind initiates the flow of ch'i, which, in turn, initiates each movement. However, each movement *intensifies* the ch'i. Thus, there is a synergistic effect that greatly escalates the flow of ch'i over time.

Sending Ch'i

An interesting phenomenon is that one person can experience and influence the ch'i of another *without any physical contact.* There are certain people who can "direct their ch'i" to another person. The other person will feel both the ch'i and a consequent reduction of the pain of an injury. It is quite a mystery how the mind of one individual can affect the ch'i of another at a distance.

My first experience with receiving ch'i that was "sent" by another was when I studied with Alice Holtman. I first met her in 1974 at a lecture she gave at the Natural Hygiene Society in New York City. The lecture was entitled, "Your Mental and Physical Stability." This title attracted me because, as a T'ai Chi Ch'uan student, I was very interested in physical stability. I felt that merging physical and mental stability would add a new dimension to my thinking. It did. At one point in her lecture, Holtman led the audience in a five-minute meditation. After the five-minute period ended, I realized that I had entered a deep meditative state. I had recently been interested in doing meditation and had tried it with no results. Now, amazingly, in a public place, under the direction of a stranger, I had experienced that which I had been seeking.

Afterwards, I asked this impressive lecturer, a short, gray-haired woman in her sixties, if she had any classes that I could attend. She replied that she was just starting a class in "Healing and Re-evaluation."

When I sat opposite her during a preliminary session, I suddenly experienced an intense tingling throughout every part of my body. I had experienced this sensation of ch'i in doing T'ai Chi Ch'uan but never throughout so much of my body or to this degree. It was so intense that I became alarmed. I scanned the ceiling, walls, and floors with my eyes to see if there was any evidence of some sort of electrical equipment that might be producing this effect. I saw nothing unusual. Then it dawned on me that the ch'i was coming from *her*. I mentioned to her what I was feeling. She replied matter-of-factly, "Good! I was sending it to you. It is healing energy. It is good that you can feel it."

The classes that followed began with a half-hour meditation. Holtman would successively focus her meditation on each student. I always knew when it was my turn because of the sudden flood of ch'i. If I then opened my eyes, I would see that she had turned and was now facing me. If I looked when I felt the ch'i abate, I would see her turning toward another student. At one point a new student came to the class. After the meditation, he exclaimed to Holtman, "I felt you beaming energy to me."

About six years later, I studied Aikido briefly with Marilyn Fountain. During one class, when a fellow student tried to throw me on the mat, I disobeyed the ground rule that students must cooperate with each other. I stiffened my arm and resisted totally. He tried again, this time using considerable force, and practically sprained my wrist. I began to rub my wrist vigorously. This was the only remedy I knew at the time. When Fountain saw this, she asked me if I was injured. I replied that it would probably recover in a few days. She said, "Let me put some ki into it." Ignoring my skepticism, she aimed the fingers of her hand toward my wrist at about a distance of six inches. Within seconds I could feel her ch'i, but it had a different quality from Holtman's. At that moment I suspected what I now know: *Each person's ch'i is unique.* Within about one minute I felt all of the pain ebb away. Then the ch'i subsided, at which time she said, "That's all it will take; it's full now." For the rest of that evening and for the next few days, I repeatedly checked my wrist by moving it in all directions and pressing it at different points. It was absolutely normal in every respect. I knew that without the ch'i, my wrist would not have recovered so quickly.

At the next class, I told Fountain how successful her ch'i treatment was. Her reply was simply, "You can do the same thing. I'll teach the class how to do it right now." In that class I learned that I had the ability to send ch'i; it was just that I never tried sending it. Of course, my studies of T'ai Chi Ch'uan and Alice Holtman's teachings paved the way for this moment.

Now, even if someone merely describes an injury, I can feel ch'i involuntarily going out from me to that person. However, I usually avoid sending ch'i unless the person's injury stemmed from my negligence. The reasons for my cautiousness will be discussed at the end of this chapter.

It is of interest that, even though I had experienced Holtman's sending of ch'i many times, I never thought to try it. I had assumed that it was a unique ability on her part rather than something anyone could develop. My lack of initiative illustrates how the *idea* of the difficulty or impossibility of something being within reach hampers its attainment.

Effect of Clothing on Ch'i

Clothing should be loose and comfortable. Also, it should be made of a natural fiber such as cotton. Synthetic fibers should be avoided.

Ch'i From Inanimate Objects

Those who are adept at ch'i can experience the ch'i of inanimate objects. Houses of worship, libraries, college lounges, and places where people regularly meditate are often strongly imbued with ch'i. This ch'i can be felt even in the absence of those who generated it.

A few years ago, I served on a committee to evaluate a certain high school. In addition to my primary role in evaluating the science facilities and program, I was asked to look over the facilities of the acting department. When I entered the theater, which was a small cathedral-like room, I saw the acting teacher sitting on the floor in the center of the room, preparing for the next group of students. As I conversed with him, I noticed an unusually strong flow of ch'i throughout my body and wondered whether it was emanating from him or from the room, itself. I decided that I might be able to feel enough of a difference to answer this question if I could get him to change his location in the room. I advanced toward him in the hope that he would not want to be that close to me and would move. However, he merely rose to a standing posture and remained at the same spot during our entire conversation about his work. Finally, in desperation, I said, "There is a lot of energy in this room." To this he placidly replied, "The Sufis use this room for their meditation every week."

Feng Shui

The Chinese use a system called *Feng Shui,* which relates the ch'i of structures to their surroundings. Elements of Feng Shui include adjacent structures, hills, trees, earth, wind, water, and roads. In traditional China, no important structure was designed without taking its Feng Shui into consideration. Here in the Western World, we erect structures with almost total disregard of their relationships with nature.

Cautions About Ch'i

Anything that has the potential to do good has an equal potential to do harm. Despite the wonderful benefits of circulating and sending ch'i, there are harmful effects. Such harm is easily avoided by adhering to the following guidelines:

1. When circulating the ch'i, no problem arises as long as the ch'i is not "forced." *Forcing ch'i* is to attempt to get the ch'i to flow in an unnatural manner. Such forcing is part of certain exercises for developing the fighting and breaking applications of ch'i. Forcing the ch'i can cause a disruption of involuntary bodily processes, resulting in sickness.[2] Therefore, it is necessary that teachers of methods that force ch'i strictly monitor students' progress and help them through any obstacles or dangers.

   However, in doing T'ai Chi Ch'uan for health, there is no need to force ch'i. The best way to cultivate ch'i for health is to attune the mind to the way the ch'i naturally flows and then improve the conditions that maximize that flow. For example, when practicing either the T'ai Ch'i Ch'uan form or an isolated Chi-Kung exercise, you should sense both the flow and blockages of ch'i. Then, experiment with deeper levels of relaxation to encourage the ch'i to flow. The persistence of your expectation that the ch'i will become stronger is all the intention that should be applied. As you begin to experience the improved natural flow of ch'i and relate that to the particulars of the movement, shape, and inner conditions that induced it, you will improve at releasing blockages. Eventually a level is attained wherein improved flow of ch'i is initiated with the mind alone.

2. Use caution when "sending" ch'i to another person for the purpose of healing. One point of view is that the more ch'i you send, the more it flows through *you* and the more benefit you receive. The other point of view is that sending ch'i can be draining. Worse, this draining can persist afterward because ch'i continues to be unconsciously sent. Both of these points of view can be reconciled in the following manner: The draining effect is thought to stem from an impure motive on the part of the sender. An egotistical involvement, for example, can lead to your sending ch'i inordinately. Rather, the motive should be a genuine desire to help another and to see all of nature in its perfection. You should regard yourself as merely a channel. If this role is genuinely felt and moderation is employed, not only will you be unharmed but uplifted and charged.

> *The universe, like a bellows, is always emptying, always full:*
> *The more it yields, the more it holds.*
>
> —Lao Tzu (Ch. 5)

3. The cultivation of ch'i, either through Ch'i Kung or T'ai Chi Ch'uan, tends to step up the sexual function. There is a tendency for the male practitioner to expend this additional sexual energy, which, instead, should be subdued and recycled. Ch'i is like fertilizer, which, when given to a plant, makes it flower prolifically. Every gardener knows that the consequent increased production of seed pods then draws energy from the plant, at its expense. It is, therefore, a common practice to prune away the developing seed pods as soon as the flowers have wilted. Analogously, it is possible for the male practitioner to channel his own sexual energy into creative faculties rather than squandering it. More will be said on this subject in the chapter on Health, Healing, and Sexuality.

To Those for Whom the Concept of Ch'i is Difficult to Accept

When I started T'ai Chi Ch'uan I had just completed a doctoral dissertation in experimental physics. I felt that concepts with no scientific basis were invalid. You can imagine my skepticism regarding the idea of ch'i. I regarded it as a feeble way to hold together an insupportable conceptual framework. However, my mental and physical rigidity began to decrease as a result of doing T'ai Chi Ch'uan. With a sequence of experiences, some of which have been related above, I gradually began to accept the idea. Now I regularly experience ch'i intensely throughout each day.

The absence of a name for ch'i in our part of the world plus a lack of scientific validation, causes the concept of ch'i to go against the grain of the average Westerner. It is best for T'ai Chi Ch'uan beginners to adopt a wait-and-see attitude. Until ch'i is experienced, it is unwise to accept it as a reality on another's say-so. It is important, however, to keep one's mind open. Once ch'i is felt, its reality will be naturally accepted.

Notes

1. Note that, in spite of their identical spellings, *ch'i* (pronounced chee) is different from the word *chi* (pronounced *jee* and defined as "ultimate") in *T'ai Chi Ch'uan.*

2. See "Ch'i Disease! How You Can Get it, How You Can Prevent it!" *Inside Kung Fu,* Vol. 19, No. 10, October, 1992.

CHAPTER 3

Basic Ideas, Concepts, and Principles

There are numerous styles of T'ai Chi Ch'uan, the most notable of which are Chen, Yang, and Wu. Each style differs from the others in certain respects. Even *within* a given style, practitioners frequently differ in their interpretations. If two versions differ, how can we determine which is correct or if both are correct?

When I was a student of William C. C. Chen, occasionally people with some understanding of T'ai Chi Ch'uan would visit advanced sparring classes at his school. Because they did not happen to see students doing the familiar movements of the form, they would erroneously think that Chen was not teaching T'ai Chi Ch'uan. Chen would then do a few movements of the form for them, purposely breaking the basic principles. At the same time, he would ask them, "Is *this* T'ai Chi Ch'uan?" When they would say, "yes," he would disagree, explaining, "Adherence to the *principles*—not the outer appearance—is the determining factor."

When in doubt, we must appeal to the basic principles. Fortunately the principles have been recorded. They are referred to as the *T'ai Chi Classics.* The T'ai Chi Classics were written in the old Chinese mode over a time period believed to span the past millennium. Comprehension of the T'ai Chi Classics requires knowledge of both martial arts and the old Chinese style of communicating through a highly abbreviated poetry. Few are able to translate the Classics into modern Chinese, and very few are able to translate them directly into English. However, a number of translations of the Classics are available in English.[1] Every student should read and re-read the Classics.

One day a classmate of mine in Cheng Man-ch'ing's school asked him the following question: "You are a master of five excellences—painting, traditional Chinese medicine, T'ai Chi Ch'uan, calligraphy, and poetry. Which one of these is the most difficult?" Cheng's answer was, "T'ai Chi Ch'uan is the hardest because it has more principles than any of the others." Not only are the principles numerous, but they require more than an intellectual understanding. They must be absorbed through consistent practice over an extended period of time.

The ideas, concepts, and principles of T'ai Chi Ch'uan are all interrelated, and they intertwine and overlap. Because they are all of great importance and difficult to prioritize, they are listed here in alphabetical order to facilitate future reference. However, those that are basic principles will be identified as such by means of section headings in *italics*.

AIR

Aside from the breathing aspects of T'ai Chi Ch'uan (see chapter 4), practitioners consider the air surrounding them to have a special significance. Movements are done in such a manner that the resistance of the air is noticed and becomes a regulating factor. There are two reasons for this: (1) In order to actually feel the effect of the air, you need to be relaxed, sensitive, and attuned. If the movements are done in a manner that maximizes feeling the air, the movements then attain continuity and gentleness. (2) Interacting with the air promotes the flow of ch'i. The sensation of the flow of ch'i is quite similar to that of the flow of air over the skin during slow movement. One should experiment with different alignments of the joints and different degrees of subtle tension to maximize the awareness of the surrounding air. This alignment and subtle tension encourage both the flow of ch'i and the awareness of this flow. For example, the practitioner can alternately gently "squeeze" and "stretch" the air between the fingers, paying attention to the effect of this. Professor Cheng used to refer to T'ai Chi Ch'uan as "swimming in air."[2]

When outdoors, the practitioner will find that the motion of the air has a subtle effect on the movement of relaxed limbs. The force exerted by the slightest breeze will cause the limbs to move differently. In the T'ai Chi Classics, Wang Tsung-Yueh says: "A feather cannot be added, and a fly cannot alight."[3] In other words, the body must be so sensitive and delicately poised that the weight of a feather will be felt, and an insect alighting will set the whole body into motion.

BALANCE

It is not uncommon for people to say, "I would not be good at T'ai Chi Ch'uan because I have such poor balance." This implies that balance is an inborn attribute that cannot be learned or improved. Nothing could be further from the truth. Early in life, we all are unable to stand for more than a few seconds without falling. Physical balance is clearly an acquired skill.

Unfortunately, because of our goal orientation, we incorrectly tend to think that things that are *slowly* learned are *impossible* to learn. Moreover, we tend to avoid any learning activity that highlights our limitations and defects. In fact, *we gain the most from studying our areas of weakness.* Success at T'ai Chi Ch'uan is measured in terms of the process of self-improvement and its benefits rather than in terms of one's outward ability at a given time. Those who uncover their poor balance and improve it using T'ai Chi Ch'uan may achieve a more substantial improvement than those whose balance is good to begin with.

Physical Stability of Inanimate Objects. To understand balance, let us first consider, from the point of view of physics, the stability of *inanimate physical objects.* Later we will discuss the physical stability as well as the emotional stability of people. Physical and emotional stability are related.

The *Stability* of a physical object refers to its tendency to return to its initial position after being displaced. Equilibrium is the scientific word for balance. When an object is in equilibrium,[4] all of the forces acting on the object are in balance. For example, when a book rests in equilibrium on a level table, the downward force of gravity is exactly balanced by the upward force of the table on the book.

There are three types of equilibrium: stable, unstable, and neutral. To understand the distinction between the three types of equilibrium, consider a cone placed in different orientations on a level surface. First imagine that the

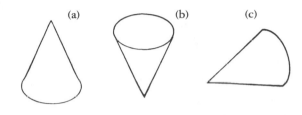

Fig. 3-1. *The three types of equilibrium. (a) stable equilibrium, (b) unstable equilibrium, and (c) neutral equilibrium.*

cone is placed on its base (see Fig. 3-1a). If it is tipped slightly, the cone will return to its initial position. This case illustrates stable equilibrium. With difficulty, it is possible to balance the cone on its apex without its falling; here, any displacement from this position will cause it to fall (see Fig. 3-1b). This case illustrates unstable equilibrium. Last, if the cone is placed on its side, any displacement will cause it to roll (see Fig. 3-1c). This case is called neutral equilibrium because it is neither stable nor unstable.

All of the postures of T'ai Chi Ch'uan should involve stable equilibrium, and the transitions should involve neutral equilibrium. In push-hands practice, the goal is to induce one's partner to be in unstable equilibrium.

The concept of center of mass is useful in analyzing balance in T'ai Chi Ch'uan. The center of mass of an object is a point that will always be directly below whatever point from which the object is suspended in stable equilibrium.

In general, the center of mass of an object whose mass is uniformly distributed is its geometric center. For example, the center of mass of a uniform rod is at its midpoint.

There are some objects whose shape is such that the center of mass is not located on the object. For example, the center of mass of a hoop is its center, at which point there is no material. In order to balance the hoop at its center of mass, we must imagine some sort of massless but rigid connection of this point to the material region.

The rule that determines the type of equilibrium of an object may now be stated in terms of the center of mass:

If any small displacement of the object from equilibrium causes the center of mass to rise, it is in stable equilibrium. If any small displacement of the object from equilibrium causes the center of mass to lower, it is in unstable equilibrium. If any small displacement of the object from equilibrium causes the center of mass to remain at the same level, it is in neutral equilibrium.

The reader should now examine the examples of the cone in each of the types of equilibrium in terms of the above rule.

Physical Stability of People. The body center, or more precisely, the center of mass of a person is called, in Chinese, the *tan t'ien* (pronounced *dan tyen*), which "... is located 1.3 inches below the navel ..."[5] and about one-third of the way from front to back. Most practitioners regard the tan t'ien to be the primary region where ch'i accumulates.

When you balance stably on one leg, your center of mass is, of necessity, above a point on that foot (ideally, that point is its center). As you bend your leg more, the center of the pressure distribution on the weighted foot tends to move forward. Similarly, when you turn to one side, the center of the pressure distribution tends to move to that side. When you waver slightly forward, the ball of the foot and toes tend to press down on the floor, and when you waver slightly to the side, the metatarsal on that side tends to press down. These corrections prevent your c.m. from extending over your base (the 100% weighted foot).

To achieve optimal stability, it is necessary to sense minute variations from center and make immediate adjustments. Instead of permitting the center of the pressure distribution to move to the front, back, or side of the foot, keep it always at center. A certain amount of practice is required to feel this centering. An exercise for precisely locating the centers of the feet will be described in Chapter 8 under "Exercises for Improving Balance."

When your weight is distributed between both feet, the center of the pressure distribution on each foot must be likewise centered on the sole of that foot. In this case, your c.m. will be directly over a line joining the centers of your two feet. Stability will be greatest along the line joining the centers of the feet (long axis of base). Conversely, stability is least in the horizontal direction perpendicular to this line (short axis of base). Therefore, in a symmetric, 50-50 stance (half of the weight on each foot), stability is poor in the forward or rearward direction.

The relationship of the human body to gravity and its surroundings is constantly changing during movement. Moreover, the human body consists of parts whose interrelationship is infinitely variable. Therefore, during movement requiring balance, the sensory apparatus and nervous system must be constantly active and are thereby improved. The challenge of maintaining one's balance while doing the T'ai Chi Ch'uan form develops the ability for the practitioner to "be in the moment."

How We Sense Imbalance. There are three ways that we sense our imbalance. One of these is visual. When we move in one direction, objects in our range of vision seem to move oppositely. Observing this apparent movement of surrounding objects serves as a sensitive indicator of whether we are wavering from a balanced position. Next, the semi-circular canals of the ears provide a highly specialized mechanism for balance. These canals, which play no part in hearing, form a three-dimensional coordinate system that sends neural messages to the brain whenever rotational movement occurs in any plane. These messages are then processed by the brain to give a perception of that movement.

The third way that we sense imbalance is through changes in pressure of the ground or floor on the soles of the feet.

Balance is perfected by attuning the above three sensory systems to even the slightest deviation from perfect balance. During each step in the T'ai Chi Ch'uan movements, the practitioner avoids committing the weight to the stepping foot but, rather, strives to be rooted and stable. As soon as balance is disrupted, the practitioner must relax and settle into a more correct alignment with respect to gravity. Balance improves as the practitioner becomes more sensitive, more efficient at the processing of sense data, and more able to relax. In short, balance improves with practice.

For specialized exercises for improving balance, see chapter 8, "Ways of Practicing."

The Effect of Others' Actions on Balance. In practicing T'ai Chi Ch'uan in a group, we often see that each person's physical balance is affected by another's movements. When one person loses his balance, others tend to lose theirs in turn. In push-hands, the object is to cause your partner to be off balance by exerting a minute but unsettling force or by subtly threatening to exert such a force. Therefore, it is of utmost importance that T'ai Chi Ch'uan practitioners cultivate a state of balance *independent of the actions of others.*

Mental Stability. Many people primarily base their ideas, behavior, morals, opinions, and perceptions on those of others. From an early age on we are exposed to the powerful influences of parents, friends, television, movies, and schooling.

While the physical practice of T'ai Chi Ch'uan predominantly involves the cultivation of physical stability that is independent of the movements of others, practitioners should similarly strive to cultivate a corresponding emotional, behavioral, spiritual, and perceptual stability.

Balancing of Left and Right Sides. While human beings are bilaterally symmetric, the two sides of our body differ in some respects. The heart, liver, appendix, spleen, and stomach are each on one side only. Moreover, many of us prefer using one side of the body to do certain tasks involving strength or dexterity. There is some evidence that the two sides of the brain differ in function. The question arises to what degree should we cultivate both sides of the body equally.

I once asked a house painter if he used both hands equally. He replied, "When I applied for my previous job, a condition of my employment was whether I could 'cut in' with either hand. When you are standing on a high rung of a ladder, it is much less time consuming to switch hands while painting than to move the ladder."

I also asked a similar question of a mason who was mixing cement with a shovel. He said, "I could not last the day if I did not switch sides."

Over the past two decades, I have experimented with using the unaccustomed side of my body for tasks or activities such as swimming, using hand tools, sharpening a pencil, peeling an orange, shoveling snow, painting, or sweeping. At first, these tasks were very awkward on the unaccustomed side, and I automatically switched back without thinking. However, after a short time, both sides equalized to the point where I even forgot which was the "preferred" side.

For example, while swimming, I realized that I always did the side stroke on one side. When I switched, it was a strange feeling to put the other side of my face in the water and to switch the roles of the left and right limbs. Soon, however, it felt natural to do the side stroke on either side. I realized that the side stroke can be done in four different ways—on each side with either version of the scissors kick.

The two-person (San-Shou) form has two roles, A and B. Recently, I taught this form to a group of my classmates under my present teacher, Harvey I. Sober. The two roles involve different movements and some of the same movements in mirror image. In his wisdom and to my initial skepticism, Sober insisted that students were to become equally proficient at both roles and learn both concurrently. They succeeded. This balanced method of learning had a fringe benefit of doubling the number of possible student combinations during practice.

When an action is known on one side of the body, it is easier to transfer this knowledge to the other side than to learn that action anew on that side. Moreover, excessive use of one side tires that side and, consequently, limits the practice time of an action. Thus, efficiency of learning is gained by using both sides more equally.

The main benefit of balancing both sides, however, is mental. Equalizing both sides of the body helps to balance both sides of the brain. Giving equal emphasis to the other side of the brain enhances the thought process. The importance of balancing both sides of the brain is starting to become recognized by psychologists.

While it is good to give both sides of the body "equal time" when doing musculoskeletal activities, a different idea applies to activities for the cultivation of ch'i. Since the flow of ch'i is not the same on both sides of the body and since the movements of T'ai Chi Ch'uan are designed to cultivate ch'i, there is a warning against doing these movements on both sides. More on this subject is contained in chapter 8 under "Ways of Practicing."

CENTERING

T'ai Chi Ch'uan cultivates (a) an ability to move in such a manner that the joints of the body are near the center of their range of movement and (b) an awareness of whatever vulnerability accompanies a departure from center. When a body part is at an extreme of its natural range of motion it is easily damaged by a small further motion. Moreover, the maximum efficiency of movement is possible only when extremes are avoided. It is an obvious self-defense mistake to place a limb in an extreme position, thus inviting an opponent to break it. In daily life, an unnaturally placed limb can be easily broken during a fall or an accident involving an automobile or other machinery.

The probability of an injury occurring from improper alignment increases with the degree and length of time that joints depart from center. Because it is impossible to continually keep joints centered, it is crucial that we build an awareness of their vulnerability so that we can come back to center when required. An analogy used by one of my movement teachers, Don Becque, was, "Once you know where you live, it is permissible to venture away from home—but not until then." Alignment is discussed more fully in chapter 5.

Another important reason for centering joints is to cultivate the natural flow of ch'i. Ch'i is obstructed to the degree that a joint is out of center. Professor Cheng emphasized what he called the *beauteous hand,* by which he meant that the wrist and fingers of the hand should have a shape resembling a line that an artist would draw.[6] The space between the fingers determines this flow to a great degree. "Squeezing" and "stretching" the air between the fingers, as previously discussed in the section on "Air" earlier in this chapter is really a way of centering the joints of the hand. The resistance felt actually stems from the natural tension of the relaxed muscles of the fingers as they move slightly away from the centered alignment.

Finally, the idea of centering of our own body parts can be extended advantageously to other actions. Excesses of all types should be avoided. For example, when you drive a car, it is a good idea to be aware of the space between your car and other cars. People who are in a hurry tend to lose their sense of proportion and endanger both themselves and others on the road. Many drivers are in the habit of repeatedly moving the steering wheel back and forth, each time over-correcting for the normal variations in the car's movement away from optimal. In most cases this unnecessary movement is merely unpleasant. However, on a slippery road surface, overcorrecting can lead to a loss of control of the car. A similar statement applies to the habit of a "nervous foot" on the accelerator pedal.

In the case of human relations, it is best not to go to extremes in dealing with others. Over-reacting can lead to conflict, which, on a world-wide scale, can be the cause of war.

Ch'i

Because ch'i is of fundamental importance and is a discipline in its own right, chapter 2 has been entirely devoted to it.

Circles

The shapes in the T'ai Chi (yin-yang) symbol are all circles (see Fig. 1-1). There is an encompassing, outer circle; two interconnected, inner semicircles that divide yin and yang; and one small circular region of opposite polarity in each semicircle. One would therefore correctly expect that circles are basic T'ai Chi

Ch'uan concepts. The circle manifests the cyclic, continuous change and interchange of nature.

The T'ai Chi Ch'uan movements involve both straight lines and circles. The final part of each move involves a strike, which, for the purposes of transferring maximum force, must be straight. However, the transitional part of each move involves a circular deflection. There are three practical self-defense advantages of circular deflections: (1) The circle has a constantly changing direction, which gives it a less predictable quality than a straight line. (2) The circle allows a large motion in a small space, maximizing the effect of an action. (3) Circular motions have a centrifugal effect that allows a deflection away from center to occur with less applied force. Moreover, the centrifugal effect is very stimulating to the flow of ch'i.

T'ai Chi Ch'uan practitioners should pay special attention to the circularity of the transitions. A common error is for the practitioner to fail to synchronize the shifting of the weight, the turning of the trunk, and the movement of the arms. For example, in the move "Rollback and Press," the left arm executes an upward circular movement, which, if the weight is shifted forward prematurely, becomes angular rather than circular in space. Care must be taken that the forward shifting of the weight starts as the left hand reaches the vertical part of its circular motion. Other moves, such as "Cloud Hands," "Brush Knee," "Single Whip," and "Looking at Fist Under Elbow" have essentially the same features.

CONCENTRATION

Concentration is the ability of the mind to become unified in its purpose for an extended period of time. It is said that the ability to *truly* concentrate for as long as one minute takes a fairly high degree of development. Why is concentration important, and why is it so difficult?

Concentration is a prerequisite to any type of creative endeavor. The word *concentrate* implies to enrich or make more rich in essence. That is exactly what mental concentration is about. When thought processes are scattered, the creative result is diluted. Accomplishing anything of value requires mental focus, and any inefficiency in this focus reduces success. For anyone pursuing a creative endeavor, the development of proper concentration is essential.

Unfortunately, the untrained mind tends to flit from one thought to another, without much conscious control. Why is concentration so difficult to develop? One possible reason is that we inwardly know that whenever we set out to do any task, we must use the time efficiently. However, because we tend to be goal oriented, we mistakenly think that the best way to use the time is to do more than one thing at a time. For example, if we are cleaning the house, we may be also thinking of many other things simultaneously such as how we will rearrange the furniture. It might even happen that the cleaning might be interrupted by trying a slight variation in the position of a few pieces of furniture. Next, a tear might be noticed in the upholstery of an armchair, and some time might be spent in seeking out a needle and thread of a certain color to mend the tear. The quest for a needle might awaken the realization that another article needs mending. And so the attention might be diverted from one task to another completely different task. The result of our skipping from one task to another is that we accomplish less than if we had done only one thing.

On the other hand, we may get a valuable idea about furniture arrangement while cleaning, but we rigidly reject this idea just because we decided to clean house and not rearrange the furniture. Thus, we might not pursue a valid direction. This example is similar to the seeming paradox of directing our own mental processes: How do we concentrate without becoming so fixated in our thoughts that the very purpose of our concentration—creative use of mind—is lost? To answer this question, let us go back to our analogy. The decisions to move the furniture and then to mend the tear, etc., should be just that: *decisions*. At each point we should be aware that we are departing from our original purpose and weigh whether or not this departure is a good idea. If it is, then go ahead. If not, then go back to cleaning. With the mind, there should be an awareness that one is drifting from a train of thought, and a decision must be made whether or not this should occur. Concentration is *not* fixation but involves a higher dimension of viewing a thought process to ensure that it is productive rather than scattered.

Just as with any endeavor, with conscious practice, concentration becomes automatic and requires less and less effort for it to proceed correctly and smoothly. Self-discipline must initially be employed for concentration to become natural and effortless. Of course, the practice of the T'ai Chi Ch'uan form is an excellent medium for the development of concentration.

CONTINUITY

> *In discontinuity there is continuity.*
>
> —Wu Yu-Hsiang[1]

The T'ai Chi symbol primarily depicts the balance of yin and yang. However, the *continuity* of the alternation of yin and yang is also depicted. Each of the qualities, yin and yang, evolves one into the other in a smooth and *continuous* fashion. After all, what could be more continuous than the circle?

A fundamental precept of science is that there are no discontinuities in nature. Scientific explanations of phenomena always leave room for the insertion of extra causal links, thus supporting our intuitive sense of the continuity of nature. When there appears to be a discontinuous change, we always seek to look deeper to uncover and fathom the missing links. A good example of "continuity in (seeming) discontinuity" appeared in the science section of *The New York Times*, October 15, 1991: "A viper's strike may only take a fraction of a second, but in this snatch of time the snake picks up with its forked tongue a distinct signature of the creature. The few odor molecules are conveyed from the tongue to a pair of sensory organs called vomeronasary glands, located on the roof of the viper's mouth, creating a chemical memory. The envenomated animal is allowed to wander off and die, but the viper can track it down wherever it may stumble." The seemingly discontinuous strike of a snake is explained in terms of a continuous succession of events.

Continuity is important in every endeavor in life. It is the expression of the philosophy of "Being in the Moment." Gaps in continuity of actions stem from gaps in mental concentration and in attunement with nature and its processes. While doing the T'ai Chi Ch'uan movements, the practitioner cultivates the mental faculties that result in continuity of action. The material for this cultivation is at hand: one's own body. The mental faculties that are developed can then be extended to other actions or ideas.

DOUBLE WEIGHTING

Double weighting is a term that is important to understand and needs explanation. Normally, double weighting is considered a fault.

Double weighting occurs when a force exerted by a person on an external object or another person is such that the reaction[8] to that force tends to uproot the person exerting the force.

Examples of Double Weighting. Consider the 50-50 stance,[9] with both feet parallel and the weight equally distributed. If a person in this stance exerts a forward force, the reaction to this force will cause the person in the 50-50 stance to lose balance and tend to fall backward. Here, equilibrium is unstable in the forward direction but quite stable in the sideways direction.

Try the following experiment. Have your partner (B) stand in any stance. Next, gently push B horizontally, in a direction perpendicular to the line joining B's feet. You will find that if B does not depart from the stance, only a very small force will be required to cause B to become unbalanced.

It should be noted that in the 50-50 stance, it is hardest to redistribute the weight between the two feet.

Note: Even though the practitioner does not exert any force on another person while doing the movements of the solo form, the potential to exert such a force is implied. Therefore, a posture or stance in a solo form can be characterized as double weighted.

DRAWING SILK

Doing the T'ai Chi Ch'uan movements is likened to "drawing silk." This simile has two different but mutually consistent interpretations: (1) In reeling silk from a cocoon, it is essential that there be no interruption in the continuity of the process; otherwise the strand will break. (2) In painting (drawing) on silk, any hesitation in moving the brush will cause an unevenness in the width of the line because of the absorbency of the silk. In either case, the underlying idea is the importance of continuity of movement.

GRAVITY

The famous "Riddle of the Sphinx" was: "What walks on four legs in the morning, two legs during the day, and three legs at night?" We start life unable to overcome gravity, and therefore we crawl. Later we overcome gravity to the extent that we walk upright on two legs. Toward the end of our lives, we start to lose this battle and need to walk with a cane. Practitioners soon realize that T'ai Chi Ch'uan builds the strength of the legs to an enormous degree. Consequently, elderly practitioners do not easily succumb to gravity.

Aside from its strength-building aspects, T'ai Chi Ch'uan deals with gravity in a number of other important respects. Because the motions are done using the minimum tension, gravity becomes an important force for which to compensate. The force of gravity has the important characteristic that it is constant in magnitude and direction. Gravity is, therefore, dependable and completely predictable. Thus, gravity is an excellent tool for studying the manner in which the body optimally deals with force in general.

Scientifically, *gravity* refers to the fact that every object near or on the Earth experiences a force toward the center of the earth. The force of gravity on an object is also called its *weight*.

One of the ways that gravity enters into T'ai Chi Ch'uan is that it assists the alternate sinking and rising of the ch'i. The movement of ch'i is related to gravity. The human body is mostly water, which develops pressure gradients because of gravity and undergoes small displacements. When we tense our muscles excessively, we restrict this movement and lose sensitivity to any subtle changes that occur. When the body attains a state of inner relaxation (sung), the internal effect of gravity during movement becomes important.

Different internal stresses occur for each orientation of the body with respect to gravity. For example, a hand tends to feel "swollen" when it hangs in its lowest position. This sensation is partly a result of increased blood pressure in that hand. However, the effect also stems from the internal pressures of gravity on the individual cells, which are slightly distorted and displaced downward. When the hand is higher than the elbow, the flow of blood and displacement of the cells is still downward but now is reversed with respect to the arm.

As the various parts of the body are moved, the internal pressures and displacements change and can be felt. Regulating the tension in a subtle manner enhances this effect, and excessive tension obstructs it.

The natural changes within a properly relaxed body serve as a kind of internal massage that is very stimulating to the flow of ch'i.

LEVELNESS OF MOTION

The T'ai Chi Ch'uan movements should be done with the top of the head at an even level. Exceptions are movements such as "Descending Single Whip," which are intended to be done at a different level. One reason for maintaining a constant level is that energy is wasted with each departure from level.

The most common error is for students to rise when shifting the weight 100% onto one foot. When the weight is shifted 100% onto one foot, it is actually necessary for the knee and ankle to bend more than in a stance in which the weight is shared between both feet.

LEVERAGE

Archimedes (287?–212 B.C.) discovered that it is possible to multiply force by means of a lever. A good example of a lever is a claw hammer used to pull a nail out of a board. The Chin Na grasping, trapping, locking, and escaping techniques utilize leverage. Sadly, many of us damage our own joints with the leverage caused by improper alignment. Alignment is treated in detail in chapter 5.

MACROSCOPIC AND MICROSCOPIC MOVEMENT

Macroscopic movement involves the motion of major body parts, all the cells of which move proportionately or essentially in unison. This coordinated movement characterizes most sports and athletic activities. For such activities, there is usually a high degree of muscular tension involved, and this tension maintains the cells of the moving parts in essentially constant relation to each other.

Microscopic movement involves the independent motion of individual cells. In the chapter on Ch'i (chapter 2), it was theorized that nutrients are transported to the cells, wastes are eliminated by means of coordinated undulations of the cells, and this undulation is experienced as a flow of ch'i. The associated microscopic movement occurs spontaneously and naturally but can be heightened in a number of ways. One of the most powerful means of heightening microscopic movement is through macroscopic movement of the correct speed, connectedness, shape, and degree of tension. The subtly tense T'ai Chi Ch'uan movements are designed to encourage this beneficial cellular movement.

"Seek stillness in motion. (Seek motion in stillness.)" This often-quoted saying can be interpreted in terms of macroscopic and microscopic movement. In order to activate the flow of ch'i, subtle outer movement is required. However, when the outer movement subsides, the fruit of this movement—the inner movement— is maximized.

NEWTON'S FIRST LAW

According to Newton's first law (also known as Galileo's principle or the law of inertia):

In the absence of any external force, if a body is at rest, it will remain at rest, and, if a body is moving, it will continue in constant motion in a straight line.

It should be noted that external forces that balance each other are equivalent to a zero external force. Thus, it may be added that when an object is at rest, the forces on it are either absent or in balance (zero *net* force).

Newton's first law is very difficult to comprehend even hundreds of years after it was first proclaimed by Galileo. One reason for this difficulty is that we seldom see a situation in which there is zero net force on a moving object. Usually there is an unbalanced force such as friction, which slows a moving object.

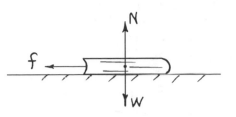

Fig. 3-2. *The forces on a book sliding to the right on a level table. W is the force of gravity on the book, N is the force of the table on the book, and f is the force of friction.*

Consider the case of a book sliding to the right on a horizontal surface and eventually coming to a stop (see Fig. 3-2). Here there are three forces acting on the book: (i) the force *W* of gravity, which pulls the book to the center of the earth; (ii) the upward force *N* of the horizontal surface on the book (this force keeps the book from falling through the table); and (iii) a horizontal frictional force *f*, which acts in a direction opposite to the book's motion and slows it down.

Because the above object remains free of any vertical motion, we can conclude from Newton's first law that the upward and downward forces balance each other. If friction could be eliminated by making the table perfectly smooth, the object would move along the horizontal surface without slowing down.

When we do T'ai Chi Ch'uan, the limbs of our body are constantly subjected to gravity. However, by using subtle muscular action, we are able to just cancel out the effect of gravity. Therefore the limbs "float" as if weightless. Moreover, as the limbs move, there is a moment-by-moment adjustment of muscular action to take into account each change of the limbs with respect to gravity. Next, if the muscular action is only the minimum required to counteract gravity, the limbs will be loosely connected to the body rather than being rigid. Then, once set into motion by the movement of the pelvis, the limbs will continue to move because of their own momentum, in a manner similar to the motion of the book on the smooth table top. Sensing this momentum is very important and is discussed in the section on "Sensitivity" later in this chapter.

Newton's Third Law

There are a number of ways of stating Newton's third law, but the following seems to be the best:

If body A exerts a force on body B, then B exerts an equal and opposite force on A.

Newton's third law is also called the "law of action and reaction." A consequence of the third law is that every time you exert any force (the *action*) on an external object or person, that object or person exerts an equal and opposite force (the *reaction*) on you.

Although the forces N and W in Fig. 3-2 are equal and opposite, they are not action and reaction. Action and reaction are always on *different* objects. Actually, the reaction to N is the force of the book on the table, and the reaction to W is the gravitational force of the book on the earth.

We do not usually notice the reactions to most of the forces we exert or feel the necessity to compensate for the effect of these reactions except in certain critical situations. For example, when we push a door open, the door pushes back on us. Therefore, we must brace against the floor. The floor, in return, exerts a reaction on us, which is a force in the forward direction that balances the force of the door. We do this bracing automatically and without conscious thought. However, if someone unexpectedly opens the door, we suddenly become aware of the reaction to the force that we exert on the floor. This force is then unbalanced and pushes us forward, causing a momentary but disconcerting loss of balance.

In push-hands practice, if force builds up between two partners, both are responsible. Neither one can say, "It's your fault."

Newton's third law can be used to great benefit because it can be used to control the force exerted by an opponent on yourself. After all, physical injuries result from sufficiently large forces. One can prevent force from building up by moving in such a manner that the opponent's attack is deflected to the side. Because the opponent braces in anticipation of a reaction opposite to the direction of the attack, it usually takes little force perpendicular to the direction of the attack to deflect it. Wang Tsung-Yueh says, "From the sentence *A force of four ounces deflects a thousand pounds* we know that the technique is not accomplished with strength."[10]

OPENING AND CLOSING OF THE THIGH JOINTS

One of the features of each of the T'ai Chi Ch'uan movements is the opening and closing of the thigh joints. These ball-and-socket joints are the largest joints of the body. Ball and socket joints allow the full range of motion: hinge action in any direction, plus swivel action. A glance at a human skeleton, model thereof, or even a picture of a skeleton, will reveal that the swivel action occurs when the knee is lifted, whereas the hinge action occurs when the knees move apart or together. The movement of the thigh joints through their full range is important for the activation of ch'i and the stimulation of glands and organs in the lower trunk of the body.

Most of the movements that we are required to do in daily life involve only a small fraction of the full range of motion of the thigh joints. In fact, moving the thigh joints through their full range is purposely avoided in polite company because it can have a sexual implication.

Consider the manner in which a person would ordinarily turn around 180° to the left, and contrast this action with that of the T'ai Chi Ch'uan form. The ordinary movement would involve a succession of several small steps to the left until the full 180° is achieved. The corresponding movement in the T'ai Chi Ch'uan form (e.g., "Single Whip") would be done by first shifting the weight 100% onto the left leg, rotating the right foot 90° to the left on its heel, then shifting the weight 100% to the right foot, and then stepping out 90° to the left with the left foot. The ordinary movement would involve almost no motion of the thigh joints. By contrast, the T'ai Chi Ch'uan action would involve first a substantial closing and then opening of the thigh joints.

The tendency to move peripherally (with a minimum motion of the thigh joints) even affects the movements of some experienced T'ai Chi Ch'uan practitioners. Some practitioners permit the knee of the rooted foot to buckle inward when the other foot takes a step, thus making up for a skimpy opening of the thigh joints. This buckling not only neglects the needs of the glands and organs but also places an inordinate strain on the knees and ankles.

P'ENG

P'eng is one of many Chinese words having no direct translation into English. Expansive or rising energy are terms sometimes used, usually resulting in incomplete understanding or total misunderstanding. Because it is crucial that p'eng pervade every movement, it requires the following detailed explanation.

P'eng and s'ung are yin and yang counterparts (see S'ung later in this chapter). S'ung is a high degree of alert relaxation and, therefore, yin (supportive, yielding, contractive). The result is an accompanying unified expansion, thereby balancing yin and yang. The expansion (p'eng) must not result from contractive muscular force but happen naturally. At first, your p'eng may be so weak that it will need to be supplemented by a relatively large degree of contractive force, which will mask it. Push-hands practice, properly done, will help to develop p'eng, especially if partners exert a moderate amount of force on each other. As your p'eng develops, you will have an increasingly springy but solid feel to others when they try to exert force on you.

PERPETUAL MOTION

One of my students, Neal Grossman, said, "T'ai Chi Ch'uan is the closest thing to perpetual motion." In physics, there are two types of perpetual motion devices, neither of which is considered to be possible: (1) a device that moves forever without the addition of energy and (2) a device that moves forever and, in addition, *produces* energy. While the T'ai Chi Ch'uan movements are not perpetual motion in the scientific sense, they are metaphorically so. A round of the T'ai Chi Ch'uan form seems never to stop, and afterwards, one feels as if energy were created.

The Long River. T'ai Chi Ch'uan is likened to a "long river." The rate at which a river flows is not the same at each place but depends on its depth, width, and other conditions. At certain locations, the river seems not to move at all. Though not easily observable, its motion, nevertheless, exists. Similarly, in those places where the T'ai Chi Ch'uan form appears to stop, activity and motion are nevertheless present.

Because of the steadiness and efficiency of the outwardly active part of each movement, the activity required to move from one place to another is minimized. Conversely, because energy of motion is stored during the outwardly inactive part of each movement, potential movement exists, even if it is not apparent.

In practical terms, the end (the yang part) of each movement involves a subtle tensing and focusing. The beginning (the yin part) of the next movement is then initiated by the releasing of this tension and focus. Therefore, even though there seems to be a stop, the energy of the motion is stored and is available for the next movement.

Elementary physics provides a good way of explaining the concepts just discussed. Consider two different types of physical phenomena:

Example 1. An automobile is traveling along a level stretch of road, when the driver then allows it to "coast." As time progresses the car slows down and eventually stops. The explanation for this deceleration is that friction with the air, etc., slowed the motion of the car. When the car comes to a stop, the frictional force also ceases instead of continuing to act on the car to speed it up in the opposite direction.

Precise measurements would show that after the car stopped, both the car and the surrounding air would now be slightly higher in temperature than when the car started coasting. Thus, even though the mechanical energy of the car disappeared, it now exists in a different form, namely, in the form of an increase in random motion (jiggling) of the molecules. More scientifically, collisions of the molecules of the moving car with air molecules resulted in the ordered motion of the molecules of the car to be transformed into a disordered motion called thermal energy. Because of its disorder, this thermal energy cannot easily be changed back into an ordered motion of the car. This thermal energy can be transformed back into mechanical energy only by means of some special apparatus such as a steam engine. Because the mechanical energy was converted into thermal energy, and the thermal energy is not easily accessible, physicists say that, in this example, mechanical energy is "not conserved." Not conserved here simply means that it was changed to a form other than mechanical energy.

Example 2. A ball is thrown vertically upward with a given initial speed. As the ball rises, it slows up, comes to a stop, and then falls downward with increasing speed. When it reaches the level from which it was thrown, it has almost the same speed with which it was thrown (almost because air resistance causes the ball to lose a small amount of mechanical energy).

Here, as the ball rises, its motion decreases as a result of the constant downward force of gravity. When the ball reaches the top, even though its motion stops, the force of gravity does not stop but continues to be downward, causing the ball to then move downward with increasing speed. Neglecting air resistance, the force of gravity first causes the ball to come to a stop, but then, it causes the ball to come back to the initial level with the same speed as initially. Therefore, when the ball reaches the top, the initial mechanical energy of motion is not lost, as was the case with the car when it came to a stop, but is *potentially* retrievable. Thus physicists say that, while the ball is rising, its energy of motion (*kinetic energy,* KE) is converted to energy of position (*potential energy,* PE). When the ball reaches the top, its energy is all PE. As the ball falls, its PE is converted back to KE. When it reaches the level from which it was thrown, the energy is all *KE*, as it was at the beginning.

Whenever the forces that act on a system are analogous to the force of gravity in the case of the ball, we say that the mechanical energy of that system is conserved. Another situation where mechanical energy is conserved is in the case of an elastic object such as a spring or bow. When a bow is flexed, the energy used to distort the bow is not lost but can be used to shoot an arrow.

In the movements of T'ai Chi Ch'uan, we seek to eliminate actions that dissipate the energy of motion. By "relaxing" muscles, we utilize natural elasticity to store the energy of motion. Also, by relaxing, we allow the force of gravity to assist in the downward portion of the movement.

Converting Translational Motion into Rotational Motion. The T'ai Chi Ch'uan movements are refined by means of a high degree of attunement to the momentum and natural motion of the bodily parts. Consider the movement "Brush Knee Left." That movement involves stepping with the left foot and then shifting the weight onto the left foot until the knee is on the same vertical line with the toe and has a weighting of 70%. Then, the body turns to the left until it is square with the direction of the left foot (see "70-30 Stance," chapter 7). In order to "conserve energy" in this sequence of movements, the following occurs: The weight is first shifted to the point where the left knee is just above the tip of the toe. At this point, the left leg becomes motionless. The shifting movement is then transformed into rotational movement of the body about the thigh joint, causing the body to rotate into square. In order for this transformation of translational motion into rotational motion to occur without disruption, it is necessary that motion about the left thigh joint be totally free.

Another example is that of the translational motion of the upper limbs being converted into rotational motion. Consider the end of the "Single Whip." After the weight is shifted onto the left foot, the body turns to square (the navel points in the same direction as that of the forward foot). At the point where the body changes from a shifting motion to a turning motion, the left upper arm and hand begin to rotate outward. The change of translational to rotational motion of the hands now follows an energy conversion similar to that just described for the body.

In addition to the gross mechanical motion of the body, there is an internal motion, namely, that of the ch'i. The dynamics of each movement result in a subtle alternate compressing and stretching of the tissues. Of course, for this subtle movement to occur, the body must "liquefy." Liquefaction requires (a) that the practitioner know the movements so well that it is unnecessary for him to think about which comes next, (b) that the practitioner's legs be very strong so that the weight can sink, and (c) that the movements be natural and coordinated precisely.

PRECISION

There is a tendency for students to underestimate the importance of following the principles *exactly*. Some beginners may disregard seeming "peculiarities" in the teacher's movements or alignment that the teacher may have spent years developing. The student must observe every detail manifested by the teacher, take seriously every correction given by the teacher, and do nothing casually.

> It is said, "Missing it by a little will lead {the practitioner} many miles astray."
>
> —Wang Tsung-Yueh[11]

ROTATION

There are numerous transitions within the form that involve the rotation of various parts of the body—especially the hands. Some of these rotations are obvious such as the rotation of the hand just before the completion of the "Single Whip," "White Crane," or "Embrace Tiger and Return to Mountain" postures. However, other rotations are more subtle and can easily go unnoticed. For example, there are rotations of either one or both of the hands just before completion of "Lift Hands," "Preparation," "Lean Forward," and "Brush Knee Twist Step" (to mention a few) and during the transitions of many other movements.

There are two main reasons for these rotations: (1) During a defense against a strike, the rotation of the deflecting wrist causes the striking limb of the opponent to be guided in a manner similar to the familiar way that boxes ride into the supermarket on rollers. Such a manner of deflecting interferes minimally with the opponent's force and induces him to become off balance. (2) The rotations are stimulating to the flow of ch'i.

The rotations should be done using a continuous motion that takes into account the connectedness and rotational inertia of all of the moving parts. To be done correctly, the rotational action requires a high level of concentration and consequent neurological activity. Thus, the rotations in the form also have a beneficial effect on the nervous system.

SENSITIVITY

Each of us is a consciousness, which, for a period of about one hundred years, dwells in and is connected to a physical body in the physical world. Being physically alive provides an opportunity to grow spiritually in a manner that would not be possible without this experience. Alternatively stated, the purpose of being "alive" is to come directly in touch with nature so that our consciousness can be imbued with a sense of its harmony. This requires (a) a means of directly experiencing pain when we do anything that is either out of harmony with nature or threatens to cut short our stay and (b) a means of experiencing well-being and joy when we harmonize with nature. Our capacity to experience pain as well as joy is proportional to the importance of our remaining in a physical body for the of spiritual growth.

It is possible to achieve a false sense of joy or to suppress pain that would otherwise help us to avoid wrong or dangerous paths. If we so choose, we can thwart our very purpose of being here. It is important to achieve a balance with nature so that we are neither cut off from it nor obsessively attached to it.

> *He who binds to himself a Joy*
> *Doth the wingèd life destroy*
> *But he who kisses the Joy as it flies*
> *Lives in Eternity's sunrise*

—William Blake[12]

The Taoist concept of nature includes the idea of naturalness as a principle of action. According to this concept, the way things happen when they are in accordance with nature is a manifestation of universal truth (the Tao).

When we are out of touch with nature, we still suffer the harmful consequences. However, in our ignorance, we do not connect these consequences with our actions.

In the T'ai Chi Ch'uan Classics, Wang Tsung-Yueh refers to the idea that the body must be so sensitive and delicately poised that the weight of a feather will be felt, and an insect alighting will set the whole body into motion. In order to achieve this goal, it is necessary for us to become extremely sensitive to anything that affects our pliability and balance.

Another important facet of T'ai Chi Ch'uan is the cultivation of ch'i. This process requires a high degree of sensitivity. Because T'ai Chi Ch'uan is a martial art, it is essential that practitioners interact efficiently and promptly with the intentions and minute movements of others. In this respect, the road of T'ai Chi Ch'uan is the opposite of today's trend toward extremes and their resulting insensitivity.

There are two factors that affect sensitivity. One is purely mental. The other is physiological. Each will be discussed in sequence.

The Effect of the Mind on Sensitivity. The mind has the ability to completely shut out strong incoming stimuli or to become acutely aware of minute stimuli. The ability to be aware or not is within our conscious control and can be developed at will by everyone.

The following probably sounds familiar: After some dental work, a patient discovers an unaccustomed irregularity on the surface of a tooth. Instead of forgetting about it, the patient continually feels it with his tongue. After a while, an aware-ness of the irregularity becomes so emblazoned on the patient's mind that it is as though that were the only thing in the world. If the patient had merely abstained from this sensitizing activity, after a day or so, the awareness of the irregularity would have subsided.

Conversely, most of us shut out messages that come to us through dreams and from others who try to help us.

In order to become open to new ideas, we must develop (a) the discernment to focus on vital things and (b) the willingness to shed pre-programmed responses.

> *Few are they that see with their own eyes and feel with their own hearts.*
> —Albert Einstein

A Physiological Factor Affecting Sensitivity: Weber's Law. The scientific principle that accounts for the desensitization produced by increasing stimuli is called Weber's law:

The minimum perceptible increase in a stimulus is proportional to the intensity of that stimulus.

An understanding of Weber's law is valuable in doing push-hands. When you contact someone, your ability to feel his intention, his inner tensions, and his bal-ance is reduced as the force you exert on him increases.

The following example involving the stimulus of visible light will illustrate Weber's law: Imagine that a human subject is placed behind a translucent screen. A given number of lit candles is placed on the other side of the screen, and sub-jects are asked to say whether they notice a change in brightness as additional lit candles are added. Of course, a subject cannot count individual candles but can only see a diffuse illumination resulting from the combined effect of all the can-dles. Assume, for example, that 100 candles are lit, and it is then found that a subject just notices an increase in brightness when ten additional candles are lit. It can then be predicted from Weber's law that if 1,000 candles are next lit, the sub-ject will not notice an increase in brightness until 100 additional candles are lit. That is, the minimum perceptible increase in brightness is always the same per-centage of the stimulus (here, 10%).

Weber's law explains why you are more likely to cut yourself with a dull knife than with a sharp one; the dull knife requires more force for its use. The increased muscular tension lowers sensitivity to force and, therefore, reduces control. Weber's law also explains why salary increases are usually not fixed amounts but, rather, a percentage of an employee's salary.

SEPARATION OF YIN AND YANG

One of the principles of T'ai Chi Ch'uan is that yin and yang must be separat-ed in all actions. The practitioner must become aware of the yin and yang aspects of each action and then balance yin and yang without confusing them.

In some actions, the characterization of what is yin and what is yang depends on the context. For example, in a posture for which 100% of the weight is on one foot, the supporting leg can be characterized as *full* and the other leg as *empty*. Full and empty are yang and yin, respectively. Thus, in this respect the supporting leg can be thought of as yang. Another (seemingly contradictory) point of view is that the supporting leg is inactive and would therefore be characterized as yin. Similarly, the non-supporting leg is active and, therefore, yang. This seeming contradiction between the two characterizations stems from the fact that yin and yang are relative to the quality under consideration, but, in many situations, there is more than one quality to consider.

Whether the supporting leg is thought to be yin or yang, separating yin and yang between the two legs will produce the same effect; namely, the non-supportive leg will not exert any force on the floor.

Even if the non-supportive leg is regarded as yin, it is not completely yin. If it were, it would be resting with its weight on the floor. Note that in the T'ai Chi symbol (Fig. 1-1), the yang part has a small dot of yin and vice versa. The dot of yang in the yin corresponds here to the small degree of tension required to keep the non-supportive leg from exerting pressure on the floor. Similarly, the dot of yin in the yang corresponds here to the fact that properly filling the weighted leg requires that the muscles of that leg be as relaxed as possible, so that there can be a "giving in" to gravity.

Another way of interpreting the dot of yin in the yang and vice versa, is to say that, as soon as anything is too yin, it becomes yang and conversely. For example, in push-hands, each partner participates in an alternation of yin and yang as follows: When one partner attacks (yang), the other must defend by yielding (yin). Once the attack is neutralized, the yin and yang aspects interchange, just as they do in the T'ai Chi symbol. A defender, who actively retreats in a manner that is inconsistent with the force and intention of the attack, is so yin that his action is actually yang. A yang response to a yang attack results in a loss.

Separation of yin and yang can also be utilized in daily life. For example, during a heated discussion, more than one person will try to talk at one time. It is best to listen (yin) when the other person is animated (yang). After a time, the other person will quiet down and naturally say, "What do you think?" That is the best time to speak and be heard.

SEQUENCE OF MOTION

One of the basic principles of T'ai Chi Ch'uan is that *all movements are initiated by the shifting and/or turning of the pelvis.* Those who are untrained invariably move in the opposite manner: namely, extremities first.

It is useful to imagine that one is surrounded by a viscous fluid, such as water or oil, and that every movement of the arms and legs necessitates their being "dragged" through this fluid. Of course, it is necessary that all body parts be as relaxed as possible so that their inertia and momentum can be felt at all times. The goal is to apply the minimum tension required to support each limb in each orientation. Since during movement, the orientation with respect to gravity of each limb is constantly changing, it is necessary to continually adjust the tension to be minimum. This adjustment engages the mind, thereby training it to "be in the moment" and to send subtle and constantly changing messages to the muscles via the nervous system.

SHAPE

Shape is one of the primary factors that influence the flow of ch'i and the degree to which the body can be strong with the minimum muscular contraction. For each posture in the form, there is an infinite range of different alignments of the arms, and, within this range, there is an optimal shape. Thus, it is necessary for the practitioner to engage in frequent experimentation in this regard.

The basic question is, "How do I know when I have achieved the optimal shape?" The first approximation is obtained by corrections from a capable teacher and by observing masters directly or through pictures. The arms of high-level martial artists have a rounded rather than angular shape. While it is important not to lift the elbows with tension, they should display an expansive buoyancy. The fine tuning of the shape of the arms is achieved by sensing the maximum flow of ch'i. Such fine tuning is difficult for those who do not yet know what ch'i feels like. However, attaining even an approximation to the ideal shape will hasten the day ch'i is felt.

It is suggested that practitioners isolate a movement such as "Cloud Hands" and continually repeat that movement in both directions in a stationary stance. The feet should be parallel and at least a shoulder width apart, and the knees should be bent. Since sung (see section on sung in this chapter) is as important as shape, it should be likewise emphasized. With each repetition, the movement should be halted at different points so that experimentation can be done with the shape and depth of relaxation. Then the movement can be continued. Other movements that lend themselves to right/left repetition in a stationary stance are "Repulse Monkey," "Brush Knee," "Diagonal Flying," and "The Fairy Weaving at the Shuttle."

Shape is important in the practice of push-hands. Here shape not only determines the extent to which energy can be released without contractive muscular force but contributes to a weakening of the opponent when he attempts to exert force.

SPATIAL RELATIONS

T'ai Chi Ch'uan practice develops an awareness of the constantly changing orientation of the body parts relative to each other and to their surroundings. This spatial awareness includes that of the foot positions of the various stances, the orientation of the body and its parts relative to the four cardinal and four diagonal directions of the compass, and the distancing of oneself from others while doing the form. Later, when weapons forms such as a double-edged sword or broadsword form are done, there must be an acute spatial awareness of the angle of the sword, its path in space, and its distance from objects in the room.

When doing the solo form for the first time in a particular room, you should be able to pick the best spot in the room to start the form. Or, if the space is physically limited, you should be able to appropriately compress the form to fit into the available space. Compression of the form is treated in chapter 8 under *Ways of Practicing*.

STEPPING

As with all actions in T'ai Chi Ch'uan, it is essential that stepping be done in accordance with the basic principles. This requirement is particularly difficult since, during stepping, the body must be balanced, with the entire weight on one foot. Before proper stepping is achieved, the legs must be strong, and the whole body must attain a high degree of relaxation.

Here are some of the basic principles that apply especially to stepping and, therefore, should be kept uppermost in mind:

Distinguish between yin and yang at all times. The muscular tension of the stepping limb must be released to the point where that limb is subtly connected to the rest of the body. During stepping, the supporting limb should obediently give in to the full weight of the body without "protest." Moreover, the top of the body must be relaxed rather than tense.

Wu Yu-Hsiang says, "Walk like a cat,"[13] which means that the weight is not committed to a foot before the foot is in (full) contact with the ground. Of course, this stepping is easier for a cat, which has four legs, than for a human being, who has only two legs.

All movements must be initiated by the motion of the pelvis, rather than peripherally. The movement of the stepping limb should be initiated by the pelvis and, then, only when that limb is totally "empty" (not exerting any force on the ground and free of unnecessary tension). Any step that is initiated by the stepping foot instead of the pelvis is incorrect.

During stepping, the axis of the trunk of the body remains vertical. There is a strong tendency to lean, especially in steps that open 135°, such as "Diagonal Flying."

Proper alignment of the ankle, knee, and hip joints must not be lost. There is a tendency for the knee of the rooted leg to buckle inward during the stepping of the other leg. If the thigh joints do not open sufficiently, then a step that is 90° or more can be taken only at the expense of the alignment of the knee.

Continuity of movement is never lost. If a foot is not empty just before it steps, it is considered to be "dead," which makes it necessary to move it using brute force. There are two reasons that a stepping leg becomes dead: (i)

The stepping leg is not totally empty of weight and, because of friction with the floor, does not respond to the motion of the pelvis. (ii) The stepping leg is tense, and the natural play of the joints of the leg is lost. Either of these conditions results in a loss of continuity of movement. The remedy is to distinguish between empty and full with respect to both legs. This illustrates that the concept of T'ai Chi (yin and yang) underlies other principles—in this case continuity.

Another aspect of continuity is the build-up of pressure of the stepping foot on the floor: After a stepping foot touches the floor, the force between that foot and the floor should build up *without discontinuity,* from zero to the full weight of the final stance.

Unity of movement is not lost. There is a tendency for the upper limbs to mechanically parallel the movement of the stepping leg or become dead. The motion of the upper limbs must also be initiated by the pelvis. When the limbs are so initiated, they may or may not parallel the motion of the stepping foot.

What Part of the Foot Should Contact the Ground First? The beginning student is told that when stepping forward, the heel contacts the ground first; when stepping backward, the toe contacts the ground first; and when stepping to the side, all parts of the foot touch at the same instant. *Stepping forward* refers to a step at an angle of less than 90° with the medial plane (see Fig. 7-1 for the definitions of the body planes). *Stepping to the side* refers to a step at an angle of 90° with the medial plane or, equivalently, to a step in the frontal plane. *Stepping to the rear* refers to a step at an angle of more than 90° with the medial plane.

Many beginners—especially those who have studied ballet—tend to step forward with the toe contacting the ground first. Such a manner of stepping is incorrect for the following reason: After stepping forward, the body center will shift in the forward direction. However, if the toe touches down first, the weighting of the foot will proceed from toe to heel, which is in the reverse direction (rearward). The progression of transfer of weight and the movement of the body are thus contradictory.

Experienced practitioners of T'ai Chi Ch'uan step forward by extending the empty foot until the heel touches the ground. Next they uniformly shift their weight to that foot as more and more parts of the foot successively make contact with the ground. The question arises whether or not this manner of stepping commits the weight to the stepping foot prematurely. If the weight starts to shift before the whole foot has made contact with the floor, how is the practitioner to know that there will not be an unexpected problem with the ground? For example, there might be a hole under the rest of the foot. True, if the contact of the foot is uniformly increased, the practitioner will be likely to discover the lack of footing before the weight is fully committed. However, it would be best not to commit the weight at all before full contact is made. When stepping forward, if all of the parts of the foot simultaneously touch the ground without committing the weight, the maximum information is secured at the earliest point. This is a more advanced method of stepping.

More advanced students can practice by imagining that the sole of the stepping foot is like a tripod. One point is the heel, and the other two points are the first and last metatarsals of the ball of the foot. All these three points of the foot should contact the ground at the same time.

Relaxation of the Legs. Just as it is very important that the upper body be free from unnecessary tension during the transitions, so should the lower body. During stepping, the toes, ankles, knees, and thigh joints should be loose. The stepping should have a liquid quality.

Here is an exercise that I have found to be very helpful in achieving this relaxation: Assume the "Hands Playing the P'i P'a" posture (just before the second "Brush Knee"). Here, the heel of the forward foot should just touch the ground with no pressure. Instead, for the purpose of this exercise, try first relaxing the forward leg so that it is entirely supported by the ground. Next, gradually support the weight of this foot with the minimum tension until it just reaches the "empty" stage—that is, touching the ground with zero pressure. Then, without losing this minimum-tension state, continue into "Brush Knee." Of course, any other move that starts in a 100% posture can be equally used.

By repeating this exercise, you will become much more able to connect the stepping leg with the rest of the body. When the stepping leg is empty, relaxed, and loosely connected to the rest of the body, then, and only then, will the leg automatically become air-borne at the appropriate time. Otherwise, when there is tension in the stepping leg, or when the stepping leg exerts pressure on the floor prior to stepping, the step is awkward and ill-timed.

Relaxation of the Feet. During stepping there is a tendency for the tendons in the upper part of the foot to become taut. Also, the toes tend to lift. You should release these tensions.

Walking Through Leaves. During stepping it is useful to imagine oneself walking through waist-high leaves. The image of a slight drag caused by the leaves is helpful in relaxing the lower legs and feet as they are moved by the upper legs and is helpful in relaxing the upper legs as they are moved by the pelvis. The image also facilitates the correct sequence of motion: body center first and extremities last.

The Importance of Keeping the Center of Gravity Low During Stepping. The lower the center of gravity, the larger a step it is possible to take without committing the weight.

The Importance of Additional Bending of the Rooted Knee During Stepping. If the knee does not increasingly bend as the weight is shifted 100% onto that leg, the body will tend to rotate upward as the weight is shifted. This concept must be taken into account if you are to keep an even level during stepping. The same concept also applies to the shifting of weight during transitions where no stepping occurs, such as "Withdraw and Push."

STICKING

Sticking has a number of facets.

In a self-defense situation, sticking involves maintaining physical and mental contact with the opponent. This contact, among other things, provides a sensitive indication of any change in the opponent's balance and intention.

While doing the T'ai Chi Ch'uan movements in a group, each individual practices sticking by being aware of the movements of others. In this way, the whole group of practitioners moves as a unit. Just as all of the body parts of a single practitioner should move harmoniously in relation to each other, so should all of the members of the group. There are three main benefits of sticking while doing the form as a group:

1. Sticking improves the ability to observe the timing and movements of others and to adjust accordingly. This improves attentiveness, concentration, reflexes, and awareness of the intentions of others.

2. Sticking provides an opportunity to observe subtle differences between your own movements and those of the leader or teacher. This results in an improved awareness of the shape and timing of the movements. Moreover, because the student is aware of and moving simultaneously with the teacher, it is easy for the teacher to communicate small corrections to the student without breaking the flow of the movements.

3. The necessity of observing others—even from behind—exercises peripheral vision and improves the ability to interpret sounds and minute currents of air caused by the movements of others.

STRENGTH

The use of strength in T'ai Chi Ch'uan is widely misunderstood. The misunderstanding stems from the fact that there exists more than one type of strength. The kind of strength used by most people can be characterized as *contractive muscular force.* Contractive strength occurs as a result of muscles contracting (shortening) and is the kind of strength used by weight lifters. Contractive strength is awkward, rigid, difficult to subtly adjust, and difficult to sustain for any length of time, and it results in an insensitivity to minute changes in force.

Another type of strength can be characterized as *expansive.* Expansive strength occurs as a result of muscles extending (lengthening).

Expansive strength is closely related to sung. Sung involves releasing contractive tension and liquefying and opening up the whole body. Once the body is in a state of sung, there is a consequent expansion. With repetitive practice, a degree of expansion is gradually developed to the point where, to an opponent who uses contractive strength, the practitioner's body feels like steel anchored in concrete. Expansive strength has the potential to receive the force of an opponent, store it like a spring, and release it with devastating effect.

SUNG

The Chinese word *Sung* does not translate into any single English word. Sometimes relax is used. However, our idea of relaxation of body parts excludes any tension, shape, or mental awareness. *Sung* incorporates the idea of relaxation with a subtle expansive tension and consequent aliveness that promotes the flow of ch'i and maintains an open and centered alignment of the joints.

While it may seem that relaxation is easy to attain, nothing could be further from the truth. Our tensions and blockages are so familiar to us that they are difficult to identify and, when sensed, are not easily relinquished. It is as though our very identity were embodied by these tensions, and releasing them gives us a feeling of insecurity. Moreover, giving in to gravity in a standing posture requires legs that are very strong. Thus, there are both psychological and physiological barriers to attaining sung. The lower the region of the body in which sung is to be achieved, the more the muscles of the legs "protest."

Therefore, it is best to start by releasing the upper part of the body—the face, neck, shoulders, wrists, elbows, chest, and abdomen. As the various parts release, there will be a distinct swelling feeling of the abdomen in the area below the navel (the tan t'ien). The swelling then progresses upward into the limbs, thereby inducing a feeling that they are supported without the familiar contractive tension. Later, as the legs become stronger, sung will begin to extend lower and lower. Consider a 100% posture. Here the muscles of the weighted leg are stretched to their full length. Because there is a large stress in the leg muscles, they tend to contract to protect themselves from this stress. To the extent that the muscles contract, they are not in a state of sung. To be sung, they must give in to gravity. A good analogy is that of concrete poured into a form. When concrete is poured, it should fully settle, otherwise there occur internal voids and consequent weaknesses. Similarly, it is necessary to liquefy the body so that everything inside settles without voids; that is, the inside opens so that there are no restrictions to internal settling.

Achieving sung requires legs strong enough to withstand tremendous stress without "protest." At the same time, practicing sung strengthens legs. The process of achieving sung takes time, persistence, and a willingness to withstand temporary discomfort. It is essential that correct alignment of arches, ankles, and knees be achieved before gradually allowing sung to permeate the lower legs. Any lingering pain in the knees is a sign of poor alignment or exceeding the rate at which tendons can strengthen.

In the postures of the form, sung must eventually permeate the whole body down to the soles of the feet. Any interruption in sung corresponds to an internal weakness in rooting, receiving energy, and issuing energy.

SUSPENSION OF THE HEAD

It is frequently stated that the head should be suspended as if by a string from above. This implies that the head should be buoyed up rather than simply resting on the top vertebra of the spine. When the buoyant effect is achieved, it is accompanied by a noticeable increase in the flow of ch'i.

UNITY OF MOVEMENT

All parts of the body must be lightly strung together, so that when one part moves, all parts correspondingly move. The mind encompasses and directs the movement of all parts. No part should move as though cut off from the mind or the other parts of the body.

VERTICALITY OF THE AXIS OF THE BODY

It has been my experience that unless students are instructed to keep the axis of their body vertical, they will lean forward, backward, or to the side. While it is true that in a self-defense situation it may be desirable to lean a bit, any leaning must be done as a voluntary act, not by accident. Therefore, it is essential that each student strive to be able to do the complete form without any leaning whatsoever. Even the "Descending Single Whip" can be done without leaning. In fact, doing it that way provides much more of a challenge to the practitioner to open the thigh joints.

VISION

There are two main ideologies concerning the manner in which the eyes are used. One idea is that the eyes should be involved in each action, thereby infusing it with the maximum focus and intention. Practitioners of this ideology "follow" the movements of the hands with the eyes, thereby focusing ch'i.

Other practitioners do the T'ai Chi Ch'uan movements letting the eyes scan the horizon, with the nose almost always pointed in the same direction as the navel. This latter way was emphasized by Cheng Man-ch'ing, who felt that the principle of non-intention dictates that the eyes should "see" but not "look."

Seeing involves the processing of the sense data that enters the eyes, without any preconception of what is or is not the most important. *Seeing* involves non-intention, whereas *looking* involves intention. When we look, we turn our heads and move our eyes. When we see, we allow the information to enter our eyes and expand our awareness to maximize the processing of sense data.

Taoist philosophy regards *looking* as narrowing awareness and objectivity. When the form is practiced with the head not turning and the eyes relaxed and taking in everything in the full 180-degree panorama, peripheral vision improves noticeably. Peripheral vision is more than a condition of the tissues of the eyes; it is also a function of the manner in which the brain processes the neural information.

Following the active hand with the eyes while doing the form definitely enhances the focus of ch'i. Therefore, it is good to practice both ways of using the eyes—one way to improve peripheral awareness and the other way to focus ch'i. Only one method should be used, however, during a given round of the form.

The practitioner should become expert at both methods before having any philosophical preference for either one.

VISUALIZATION

The word *visualization* refers to the forming of mental images associated with vision. When we "imagine" something, our perception is mainly visual. This is because a relatively large portion of our brain is given over to the processing of sense data from the eyes. When we understand an abstract explanation, we say, "I see." Perhaps, if we were more like dogs, whose brains are more geared to the processing of *olfactory* sense data, we would say, "I smell" when we understood.

Visualization is extremely important to the learning process. "Seeing" events in our "mind's eye" is a powerful mechanism for actuating those events and processing their consequences, without the necessity for anything to occur in the physical world per se.

When we visualize a sequence of events, our nerves carry minute impulses to the very muscles that would be involved in the imagined actions. In fact, it is believed that, during dreams, there are small muscular movements corresponding to the action in the dream (*scanning hypothesis*).[14]

A few years ago I heard a radio interview with a famous ballet dancer. He mentioned that he showed such promise as a student, that he was thrust onto the stage even before he had mastered certain basic movements. A more experienced colleague noticed this problem and said, "Spend some time every day visualizing yourself perfectly executing each move that you now find difficult." After only a few weeks, the dancer was able to do every movement without difficulty.

I recently had a similar experience. There were two stretching postures that I had avoided for years because I had such difficulty with them. One night I had a dream that I was doing both of these with perfect ease and enjoyment. The next day I decided to add these stretches to my regimen. I still am unable to do these stretches to the extent that I did them in the dream, but I have made excellent progress with them. There is no question that my dream not only gave me the incentive to work to attain the flexibility I imagined, but, it created a continuing memory of how it felt to do these stretches effortlessly. This memory has helped me to stretch more correctly. Another way of viewing this experience is that certain negative ideas I had about my abilities became a limiting factor. This limitation was then dispelled by my dream in which I saw myself accomplish what I thought I could not.

As a physics teacher for the past thirty-two years, I have seen many students sabotage their own progress with the words I can't. All thoughts and verbal expressions affect the subconscious mind, which slavishly accepts what is repeatedly said or thought. Saying or even thinking, "I can't" acts in a hypnotic fashion to negatively program the subconscious mind, greatly reducing chances for success. While we should not go overboard in the other direction by thinking that we can accomplish what is physically impossible, many things that we think are impossible are only so because of the limitations we, ourselves, impose.

When I was a beginning student under Prof. Cheng, I would watch him doing push-hands with more advanced students. At that time I did not understand what he was trying to teach. However, the visual image of what he did became engraved in my mind. Now, many years later, some of these memories shape my practice. I visualize Prof. Cheng's response to a certain push-hands situation that I encounter in my practice. I then try to do what I see him do in my mind's eye.

Visualization is used to a great extent in sports. Athletes practice by visualizing actions that they may be called upon to perform. For example, when a baseball player stands in the outfield, he visualizes himself doing the play that will be required if the ball comes to him.

A few years ago, my present teacher, Harvey I. Sober, asked me to demonstrate the T'ai Chi Ch'uan broadsword form at his yearly exhibition. I knew that there would be an audience of approximately one thousand people, many of whom were highly accomplished martial artists.

The broadsword form involves many movements that are only slightly different from one another. Moreover, because this form involves many turns, I was concerned that missing one turn would result in my ending the form with my back to the audience. To avoid this embarrassing possibility, during the weeks prior to the exhibition I mentally practiced the form at every opportunity, visualizing myself on the stage with the audience present. I even visualized the orientation of each move with respect to the audience, as well as to the curtain and the wings.

Once on the stage, I felt an overwhelming sense of energy and calm. I attribute this feeling partly to the concentration of the audience and partly to the residual energy of those who exhibited before me. However, the good feeling stemmed primarily from the fact that I had previously visualized myself in that situation so many times that I felt at home.

A good time to use visualization is when you are so sick that it is impossible to physically do the form. Not only will you progress at T'ai Chi Ch'uan, but you will also be assisting the recovery process.

Visualization in Daily-life Situations. We can extend the practice of visualization to our daily lives by (a) asking ourselves, "In what manner could I have acted in this situation such that the outcome would have been more beneficial to all concerned?" and then (b) visualizing this beneficial outcome. Practicing such a form of visualization on a regular basis increases the likelihood that future reflex interactions will be improved. It is crucial that for good results, the motive here must be for learning rather than for self-blame. Our past is a reference library, which should be used objectively and without blame.

Reviewing our mistakes is valid. However once the point is reached where we have learned all that we can from the mistake, then continued review becomes self-flagellation and sabotages our progress.

There are a number of ways that visualization can be used in a negative manner, and these ways must be avoided. In situations with people or events, negative visualization can actually promote the occurrence of the negative events that are imagined. Conversely, envisioning people or interactions between people in their perfection can pave the way for their improvement. As a physics teacher, I frequently visualize my students, mentally amplifying what I know are their best but latent qualities. At the very least, my "envisioning them in their perfection" enhances *my* expectation for their growth. However, constructive envisioning may well have a *direct* beneficial effect, which may some day be explained in scientific terms.

Notes

1. See *The Essence of T'ai-Chi Ch'uan: The Literary Tradition.*

2. See Cheng Man-ch'ing, *T'ai Chi Ch'uan: A Simplified Method of Calisthenics & Self Defense,* North Atlantic Books, Berkeley, CA, 1981, pp. 39–40.

3. *The Essence of T'ai-Chi Ch'uan: The Literary Tradition,* p. 35.

4. *æquus* (equal) + *libra* (balance).

5. Cheng Man-ch'ing, *Cheng Tzu's Thirteen Treatises on T'ai-Chi Ch'uan,* Translated by Benjamin Pang-jeng Lo and Martin Inn, North Atlantic Books, Berkeley, CA, 1985, p. 38.

6. See Cheng Man-ch'ing and Robert Smith, *T'ai-Chi,* Charles E. Tuttle Co., Rutland VT, 1967, p. 68. See also Figure 5-1 and its accompanying discussion.

7. *The Essence of T'ai-Chi Ch'uan: The Literary Tradition,* p. 58.

8. See "Newton's Third Law," later in this chapter for an elucidation of reaction.

9. See chapter 7 for a discussion of stances.

10. *The Essence of T'ai-Chi Ch'uan: The Literary Tradition,* p. 37.

11. *The Essence of T'ai-Chi Ch'uan: The Literary Tradition,* p. 40.

12. From F. W. Bateson, *Selected Poems of William Blake,* Heinemann Press, London, 1978, p. 88.

13. *The Essence of T'ai-Chi Ch'uan: The Literary Tradition,* p. 56.

14. William C. Dement, *Some Must Watch While Some Must Sleep,* W. W. Norton and Co., New York, NY, 1976, pp. 47–52.

CHAPTER 4

Breathing

EVERYDAY BREATHING

The average person takes tens of thousands of breaths per day. Nevertheless, most people pay little attention to breathing and may go a whole lifetime without ever questioning whether breathing may be improved in any respect. Such a lack of attention is a serious problem because breathing tends to become more and more shallow and ineffective from birth on. We will examine why this deterioration occurs, but first, let us analyze the process of breathing.

There are two natural and primary ways of breathing. One way involves a bellows-like action of the ribs. When the ribs move outward, the lungs expand and fill with air; when the ribs move inward, the lungs contract and expel air.

The other primary way of breathing involves a piston-like action of the diaphragm. When the diaphragm extends downward, the lungs expand and fill with air, thereby expanding the lower abdomen.

Both of these ways of breathing are natural and effective.

Unfortunately, most people use only a small fraction of their total lung capacity. This deficiency is known to those who teach disciplines such as singing, playing a wind instrument, athletics, yoga, and martial arts. Just watch people with whom you have daily contact. Notice how frequently and shallowly they inhale and exhale. Why is shallow breathing undesirable? How did natural breathing deteriorate? How can inefficient breathing be reversed? Let us treat each of these questions in turn.

The Importance of Efficient Breathing. Air is the most important of the things we depend upon for life. It is possible for most people to go unharmed without food for a month. It is possible to go without both food and water for a few days. However, almost no one can survive without air for more than a few minutes. Therefore, efficient breathing should be a matter of utmost concern. Moreover, the physical action of every breath we take causes the internal organs to be massaged and facilitates the movement of nutrients and wastes. Additionally, the muscles that are used in breathing link the upper and lower parts of the body. Such a linkage is especially important in actions that occur in athletics or martial arts, which require the efficient transmission of energy from the legs to the upper body.

For any type of spiritual discipline it is essential that sufficient oxygen reach all parts of the body—especially the brain. The inefficient manner in which most untrained people breathe is a poor compromise between receiving sufficient oxygen and the lazy rebelliousness of the atrophied muscles of the diaphragm and ribs. Furthermore, the natural motions associated with deep breathing help to open up the chakras through which ch'i (alternatively called *prana* or *ki*) enters the body. The oxygenation of the cells and the ebb and flow of natural breathing stimulate a corresponding flow of ch'i. Finally, concentrating on natural breathing frees the mind from mechanical, everyday, fixated thinking. This mental shift is a first step towards entering a meditative state.

Reasons for Inefficient Breathing. If you watch a newborn infant, you will see that its whole abdominal area is involved in the breathing process. That is why abdominal breathing is referred to as "early breathing." When the diaphragm is used for filling the lungs, it extends downward, causing the lower abdomen to swell out. In elderly people, abdominal breathing is usually absent, and only the smallest motion of their upper chest is observable. Thus, breathing that only involves the upper chest is referred to as "late breathing."

How does breathing, a function that is so essential to life, become stunted? In my opinion, it has a lot to do with clothing.

Most clothing is not designed with considerations of optimal breathing in mind. The general effect that most clothing has on breathing is as follows: When people wearing conventional clothing take a deep abdominal inhalation, they feel the pressure of a belt or waistband against their abdomen. When they breathe out fully, their clothing becomes too loose and feels as though it will slip down. People unconsciously learn that deep breathing causes inconvenience and stop breathing deeply. When I started practicing deep abdominal breathing, I found out that wearing a belt—or even loosely fitting drawstring pants—was very uncomfortable. After a few years of struggling with clothing that was either too tight or slipping down, I tried wearing suspenders. Now it would be unthinkable for me to go without them. Since I have been wearing suspenders, I have noticed that, when on "automatic pilot," my breathing has become very deep.

When dressing, I adjust the drawstring to be slightly loose when taking the most expansive breath I can. When I exhale completely, the suspenders come into play. This is a very simple solution to such an important problem!

Another factor that inhibits natural breathing is that we are living in an environment in which the air is polluted. We unconsciously feel reluctant to inhale air that we know includes the exhaust of motor vehicles, incinerators, etc. Of course, when in a heavily polluted environment it is best to avoid deep breathing. However, we must compensate for this avoidance when we are able to breathe air that is relatively clean.

It has been my experience that people who habitually inhale tobacco smoke tend to breathe in short, frequent, shallow spurts. It would appear that the traumatized lungs of these smokers have lost their ability to expand painlessly to their optimal size.

Less-than-optimal breathing may also stem from an event we have all experienced—childbirth. In childbirth, infants are suddenly ejected or forcefully pulled from the almost-perfect environment of the womb where they have grown from a single cell into a completely formed human being during a nine-month period. They are thrust from conditions of constant temperature, the buoyancy of the amniotic fluid, and the oxygenation provided by the umbilical cord. Frequently, they are immediately held upside down by their frail legs and slapped to cause them to take their first breath. Imagine the strain on a newborn child, who has developed in a virtually gravity-free environment, to be suddenly treated in this extreme manner!

When we intervene in any process of nature and impose our idea of how that process should occur, we must be very careful not to tamper with the natural rate. Rather, our goal should be to discover natural principles and extend these principles to all actions.

An obstetrician, Charles LeBoyer, has delivered thousands of infants without subjecting them to unnecessary trauma.[1] To ease the discomfort of a newborn infant, he does not sever the umbilical cord immediately, as is usually done by other obstetricians. A premature severing of the cord places the infant's life in danger and requires it to gasp for breath to receive needed oxygen. Instead, LeBoyer allows the exhausted infant to float in warm water or rest on its mother's abdomen for a while after its ordeal of passing through the birth canal. In this way, it receives oxygen from its mother until it is ready to breathe on its own. It soon breathes voluntarily and naturally. Only after the child is ready is the umbilical cord tied off and severed. The child is made comfortable and eased into the world instead of undergoing a life-threatening trauma.

There is no telling to what extent the memory of the birth trauma pervades the lives of those of us who have been delivered in the usual impatient, callous manner. Being forced to breathe prematurely may well account for the fear that many people have of exhaling fully. The sense of having no air in our lungs may revive a memory of a near-death experience during childbirth.

A Conjecture about the Direct Absorption of Oxygen to the Brain. Those who cultivate optimal breathing consider the openness of the nose to be an important factor in the efficient absorption of oxygen. I am convinced that oxygen reaches the brain and eyes, not only through the lungs and blood stream but, also, *directly*, through the nasal passages. This concept would explain why it is so hard to concentrate when your nose is stopped up and why the nostrils dilate at times of stress. The brain is an organ for which an unceasing supply of oxygen is crucial, and it is conceivable that such an important organ would have a *direct* source of oxygen.

If it is true that oxygen is absorbed to the brain directly through the nose, then it is important that the nasal passages be kept as free as possible of obstructions. Before doing meditation, practicing breathing exercises, or engaging in any demanding pursuit, it is wise to cleanse the nasal passages very gently and carefully, using water and clean hands. More elaborate methods of nasal cleansing such as netti[2] are valuable but should be initially attempted only under the guidance of an adept practitioner of this art. During practice of deep breathing, you should also strive to develop the ability to dilate the inner nasal passages to increase possible absorption of oxygen. Moreover, a conscious attempt should be made to channel the flow of air through the upper regions of the nasal passages when inhaling. In fact, if you pay careful attention to natural breathing, you will find that, during inhalation, air is automatically channeled higher in the nasal passages than during exhalation. One reason for this differentiated channeling is that the inhaled air needs to be humidified and filtered, but the exhaled air does not. Another possible reason is that the exhaled air is lower in oxygen and, if channeled through the upper passages, would *remove* oxygen from that region at the expense of the brain. By consciously channeling the inhaled air through the upper nasal passages, we are enhancing what is evidently a natural and beneficial process.

An Abdominal Breathing Exercise. There are many breathing exercises practiced by students of Yoga and of martial arts. Here is one that I have found to be of value:

Lie on your back on the floor. A bare or rug-covered wooden floor is best. In warm weather, lying on grass or sand outdoors is certainly beneficial. Stone floors are to be avoided. Cover your abdominal region with a blanket if there is any chance that you will need it. (It should be kept in mind that the air near the floor is usually lower in temperature than at waist level, and, when the body is quiet, it tends to produce thermal energy less rapidly.) First spend a few minutes relaxing every part of your body and noticing your breathing. Next, take slow, smooth, deep breaths into the lower abdomen, expanding the waist area in all directions. Even the back and sides should expand. The idea is not to hyperventilate but to take in a normal amount of oxygen in a special way, namely, by filling and emptying the lungs more efficiently. While you are breathing, let the ribs release downward during both inhalation and exhalation. (The reason for subduing the ribs is not that it is bad to use the ribs for breathing but, rather, to isolate and practice the type of breathing in which most of us are deficient.) Concentrate on the transitions between inhalation and exhalation and try to eliminate all discontinuities. Think of the breathing as following a pattern analogous to the T'ai Chi symbol, in which yin and yang evolve continuously one into the other. In breathing, there should be a smooth transition between inhalation and exhalation, with no "sharp corners." If this exercise is practiced daily for a period of time and if clothing is worn that does not interfere, abdominal breathing should become more and more automatic.

After this important first step, you should become aware of the effects of breathing beyond those involving the lungs, ribs, abdomen, nose, and throat, all of which *directly* participate in the breathing process. For example, you should start to become attuned to the effects of an inhalation or exhalation upon pain reduction, enhancement of ch'i, and whatever else occurs.

The above breathing exercise is only one of a great many valuable ones. An excellent introduction to yogic breathing is contained in Yogi Ramacharaka's book, *Science of Breath*.[3]

It should be borne in mind that the purpose of breathing exercises is to isolate and practice a particular manner of breathing that is stunted or completely overlooked. Beware, however, of picking a particular exercise and attempting to habitually breathe that way. That defeats one of the main purposes of breathing exercises—*the elimination of breathing fixations*.

T'AI CHI CH'UAN BREATHING

In general, T'ai Chi Ch'uan teachers vary in their advice to students about how to breathe while practicing the T'ai Chi Ch'uan form. Some encourage students not to think about breathing. Others give specific directions about when to breathe in and out. Furthermore, not all of those who give specific instructions agree on when to breathe in or out. Some say that the final (striking) part of the movements should involve an inhalation. Others say that the final part of each movement should involve an exhalation.

The nonuniformity of breathing patterns among T'ai Chi Ch'uan teachers is in sharp contrast to a uniformity among teachers of "hard styles," who all agree that the final (striking) part of each move should be accompanied by an exhalation and that the transitions should involve an inhalation.

My first teacher, Cheng Man-ch'ing, told us not to think about breathing. His ideas about breathing stemmed from the concept of *non-action*. Cheng was concerned that we might do ourselves harm if we contrived our breathing to follow any particular pattern. He would only tell us that the lifting of the arms in the "Beginning" posture involved an inhalation and would then say that, in the rest of the movements, the breathing would take care of itself. By telling us the natural breathing pattern of the first movement, Cheng was giving us a way of corroborating our sense of the naturalness of breathing in that movement and, therefore, in all movements.

My next teacher, William C. C. Chen, told us very clearly where to inhale and exhale. In his view, except for the "Beginning" and final "Close-Up" movements of the form, exhalations occur during transitions, and inhalations occur during the final part of each movement—oppositely to hard styles. In his book,[4] circles are used to indicate where inhalations occur. While Chen's recommendation is clearly defined, it is meant to be conscious only at first and not to be rigidly practiced. Its pattern is consistent with the natural way of breathing that would occur for a practitioner who follows Cheng Man-ch'ing's non-action approach.

My present teacher, Harvey I. Sober, has both a very extensive soft- and hard-style background. He is a master of Chen boxing, Monkey style, Crane style, Pa-Kua Ch'uan, and Hsing-I Ch'uan—as well as a Karate grand master. While Sober is capable of tremendous power and strength, he uses the legendary "four ounces" when he demonstrates T'ai Chi Ch'uan self-defense applications. He knows and teaches *many* different methods of breathing and encourages his students to become familiar and experiment with *all* of them.

A Natural Breathing Pattern. Allowing breathing to occur in an unrestricted manner will reveal that inhalations naturally occur when the arms rise, such as in the "Beginning" posture or just before the final postures of "Ward off" or "White Crane Spreads Wings." Further, exhalations naturally occur when sitting back or shifting into one leg during a transition. According to Yang Zhen-Duo,[5] the son of Yang Cheng-fu (Yang Cheng-fu was Cheng Man-ch'ing's teacher), "As for the coordination of the breath with the movement, I also emphasize a natural combination of the two. A natural combination is like this. For example, as I *fajin* (release energy and strike), because I am pushing forward and striking something at the front, I never would be breathing in. If I shift forward and at the same time I inhale, it doesn't make sense; it does not follow smoothly. If I sink downward, I really cannot inhale at the same time. Sinking and inhaling together doesn't feel comfortable. Likewise, if I do a movement that lifts upward and at the same time I exhale, it feels unnatural. Therefore, the combination of the movement with the breath must follow the natural way of the movement." Notice that Yang is not specifying a pattern to adhere to, but, rather, he is stating what feels natural and comfortable to him.

A Reconciliation of Different Breathing Patterns. The following is a synthesis of the concepts of breathing that I learned from my teachers:

The breathing done during the practice of the T'ai Chi Ch'uan movements differs from that done while practicing the movements of hard styles. In T'ai Chi Ch'uan, expansive movements usually involve an inhalation, and transitions usually involve an exhalation. In contrast, in Karate, each expansive movement involves an explosive exhalation, and each transition involves an inhalation. On the surface, these are essentially opposite methods of breathing, but, as will next be explained, while different, both obey similar principles.

In both hard and soft styles, one of the main functions of breathing (apart from fulfilling normal respiratory requirements) is to connect the upper and lower parts of the body so that energy can be directed from the ground, through the legs, into the trunk, and out of the extremities. The spine is a loosely connected series of short bone segments and is the only skeletal structure that connects the upper and lower parts of the body. The lack of rigidity of the spine results from its necessity to flex and, thereby, provide a shock-absorbing action. If the vertebrae were stacked one upon the other along a straight vertical line rather than along several curves or if the spine were rigid, then every step during locomotion would cause an impulsive jolt to the entire body. The curves of the spine allow a gentle flexing to absorb the jolts of locomotion. However, during the transmission of explosive force from the ground to an extremity, there are much larger forces on the spine than during normal locomotion. Therefore, during the mobilization and exertion of force by the upper body, the shock-absorbing feature of the spine must be increased, and a certain amount of abdominal tension is needed to keep the spine from buckling.

In hard styles, contracting the musculature of breathing provides the necessary tension and connectedness for the exertion of strength.

In T'ai Chi Ch'uan, the main idea is to cultivate the flow of ch'i and a consequent *expansive* strength. The martial aspect of T'ai Chi Ch'uan requires ch'i to be maximized in the extremities during the final (striking) part of each movement. Using contractive muscular strength not only obstructs the flow of ch'i but is awkward. Therefore, practice of the T'ai Chi Ch'uan form should not involve muscular contraction.

Because human beings locomote in an upright posture, relaxing completely would cause a person's chest and abdominal region to naturally move inward under the action of gravity, expelling air. Conversely, the natural expansion of the chest and abdomen during an inhalation requires a small amount of extensive muscular tension. Natural breathing is, therefore, the breathing most akin to the type required while practicing the T'ai Chi Ch'uan movements. Inhaling just prior to the completion of a posture involves an expansive tension (yang aspect). Exhaling during a transition involves a melting or yielding (yin aspect). During the parts of the movements that correspond to a mobilization of strength, muscular contraction characteristic of hard styles is replaced by expansive tension, which is augmented by an inhalation.

Since the oxygenation of the blood intensifies ch'i, the ch'i in the extremities tends to become greatest during an inhalation. Moreover, exhalation assists a state of sung and a consequent accumulation of ch'i in the tan t'ien. Exhaling during transitions and inhaling just prior to the finished postures is in keeping with the idea that T'ai Chi Ch'uan is an internal style whose energetics rely on ch'i rather than contractive muscular strength.

In contrast, hard styles emphasize contractive muscular strength and force. In these styles, the muscular contraction required during the striking part of each movement is large compared to that required for an inhalation. Therefore, the striking part of the movement necessitates a mode of breathing that involves a much higher degree of abdominal tension than that associated with an inhalation. Here, a sharp, explosive, voiced exhalation, called a *kiai* (pronounced *key'eye*), is frequently employed. In the transitional part of the movement the muscular tension of the inhalation is small in comparison to that during the strike and corresponds to a relative state of relaxation.

Thus we see that, although the breathing done in the hard styles is different from that done in T'ai Chi Ch'uan, the underlying principles of both are consistent. Namely, the mobilization of strength has the yang aspect, and the transition has the yin aspect. In both styles, yin and yang are accompanied by a compatible breathing pattern.

Over the past twenty years, I have experimented with different ways of breathing while practicing the T'ai Chi Ch'uan movements. At first I found that my natural inclination to breathe in or out was frequently different from my idea of "correct" breathing. However, I never attempted to force my breath into any prescribed pattern but merely noticed it. Gradually, as my mind began to encompass more facets of the movements, such as tempo and depth of breath, I found that my breathing became increasingly natural and more coordinated with the movements. At this point, I pay very little attention to my breathing, whether or not it fits any prescribed pattern. I tell my students that, in filling the postures, it feels natural for me to inhale, and, in the transitions, it feels natural to exhale. But I warn them not to contrive their breathing. Occasionally experimenting with breathing and then letting it take care of itself will eventually lead to the most desirable result.

Notes

1. See Frederick LeBoyer, *Birth Without Violence,* Alfred A. Knopf, New York, 1980.

2. See Yogiraj Sri Swami Satchidananda, *Integral Yoga Hatha,* Holt, Rinehart, and Winston, New York, 1970, pp. 174–5.

3. Yogi Ramacharaka, *Science of Breath,* Yogi Publication Society, Chicago, IL. 1904, (ISBN 0-911662-00-6), available from Wheman Bros. Hackensack, NJ.

4. William C. C. Chen, *Body Mechanics of T'ai Chi Ch'uan,* William C. C. Chen Publisher, New York, NY, 1973.

5. Yang Zhen-duo, *Traditional Yang Family Style Taijiquan,* A Taste of China, Inc., 111 Shirley Street, Winchester, VA 22601, 1991, p. 4.

CHAPTER 5
Alignment

There's nothing wrong with your body; it's the way you are wearing it.
—Elaine Summers

What is Alignment, and Why is it Important?

Alignment is the manner in which the bones of the body line up with one another. Correct alignment is important for the following four reasons:

1. Correct alignment of bones reduces stress on the ligaments, which are bands of fibrous tissue connecting two or more bones. Ligaments maintain the integrity of each joint.

   Ligaments are very strong. When alignment is good, ligaments can usually withstand the stress caused by the normal movements of everyday life. However, when alignment is faulty, a sudden external force on the malaligned joint can harm the ligaments. Here is how this harm occurs:

   Healthy cartilage can support tremendous pressure but is very slippery. When the alignment of a joint is correct, there are no lateral forces—only harmless compressive ones. Faulty alignment, however, results in harmful, opposing lateral forces (shearing stress). Because cartilage is so slippery, shear can cause an uncontrolled lateral sliding that stretches the ligaments beyond their limit. Consequently, sudden movements of a malaligned joint under abnormal external stress can result in a sprain, which is the stretching and/or tearing of the ligaments. While controlled movement of incorrectly aligned joints does not, itself, cause a sprain, habitually incorrect alignment increases the probability that the joint will be in a vulnerable state should an abnormal stress occur.

   The weight-bearing joints of the knees and ankles are especially prone to becoming sprained, and, for these, correct alignment is of primary importance. However, other parts of the body, such as fingers, wrists, and elbows can likewise be sprained if a sudden stress occurs. This stress can result from an unexpected situation such as a fall. Or, it can result from large forces applied by another practitioner during self-defense practice. Finally, it can result from an actual self-defense situation. In real (or practice) fighting, the opponent attempts to inflict real (or potential) harm on the joints. An important system of trapping and locking the opponent's limbs, called Chin Na, is based on a knowledge of anatomical weaknesses of the joints. It is therefore imperative that those who study self-defense learn the neutral alignment of every joint and the corresponding vulnerability of departures from center.

2. Chronic malalignment of joints results in unnatural pressures on regions where the cartilage is thin. These pressures can cause the cartilage to deteriorate. Ultimately, this deterioration can lead to serious joint problems, including arthritis. Sometimes the harmful effects of such a stress may not appear until years later.

3. Incorrect alignment blocks the flow of ch'i. Ch'i flows to the greatest degree when joints are relaxed and near their neutral (centered) alignment.

4. Correct alignment maximizes the effectiveness of the muscles and explains why a muscular person can be overcome by someone who is much less muscular. The reaction to the force exerted by the person on an external object or another person acts to move malaligned joints even further away from center. The tension required to keep these stressed joints from pain and damage occurs at the expense of accomplishing the task at hand.

Why is it Necessary to Study Alignment?

When we were very young, even before we were able to walk, we observed much that was around us. By the time we were ready to walk, we had already developed a concept of alignment based on that of others. As we got older, we copied the physical patterns of those whom we admired for certain things *other than* bodily efficiency. Unfortunately, during the formation of our own body identity, we may have adopted others' faulty postural and movement patterns.

A number of physical factors hamper our learning correct alignment. One such factor is clothing and footwear. As infants, we wore diapers and clothing that restricted and inhibited natural movement. Soon we were given shoes. Unfortunately, most footwear is designed more for protection, hygiene, and appearance than for locomotion (see chapter 9 for a discussion of footwear). Next, we used furniture such as desks and chairs. Furniture is frequently designed without any real attention to the physiological needs of a human body.

Another factor regarding alignment is that our emotions, tensions, sorrows, etc., tend to become embedded in our musculature. Many systems of psychology, physiology, and massage incorporate the idea that our habitual movement patterns and postural fixations echo prior emotional traumas. We all know that body movements are used to convey our emotions of the moment. Is it too far-fetched to think that accumulated traces of intense past experiences remain and are later manifested?

Still another factor regarding the use of joints is ignorance of or serious misconceptions about the anatomical details of our bones, organs, etc. This lack of understanding prevents us from correctly interpreting pain that occurs when we damage or improperly use our joints. On this point, the late Moshe Feldenkreis, a world-famous physiotherapist, maintained that some people become literally crippled as an eventual result of such misconceptions.

The following anecdote will serve to illustrate the importance of understanding proper anatomical relations:

Recently, when I was on the check-out line of a supermarket, the young woman who was "bagging" remarked to the cashier, "My knees are killing me." I involuntarily looked at her knees and saw that she was severely hyper extending them (forcing them backward). I have had a few students whose prior chronic knee problems resulted from habitual hyperextension. These problems promptly left when this habit was eliminated. I asked her if the pain could possibly result from jamming her knees back. She replied, "That's the way I always stand. My knees hurt from my exercise class this morning." Because she had no idea of the correct alignment of the knee, she was unable to relate the pain to anything over which she had control and, instead, blamed exercise.

Studying alignment based on anatomy and physiology gives us a factually grounded framework for learning about ourselves. Eventually, through educated experimentation, we can confirm theoretical principles of alignment by experiencing them. When anatomical relations are clearly visualized, we can detect and respond to murmurs for help uttered by our joints at an early stage of harm. Through practice of T'ai Chi Ch'uan, we can program correct alignment into our spontaneous movement.

Obstacles to Reversing Faulty Patterns

Over the years that I have been teaching body movement, I have encountered many students with faulty alignment and its consequent injuries. Unfortunately, old, incorrect habits feel "right," and new, correct patterns feel "strange." When people are corrected, they often say, "But this is the way I stand" or "This is the way my body is built." I reply, quoting Elaine Summers, "That is the way you are *wearing* your body" (which has two meanings). I go on to explain that it is very difficult to be objective about things you have done a certain way for many years. After a reasonable amount of time, however, the body, itself, will tell you whether or not the new way is correct.

A Personal Story

At the time when I was a beginner in T'ai Chi Ch'uan, I sprained my knee during a highly spirited game of paddleball. After a few weeks I had recovered sufficiently to walk without much pain. However, even after three years, the injury had not completely healed. My knee would ache at night, and certain movements would be painful during the day. I always had to be careful not to re-injure the knee in doing the form, push-hands, or sparring.

About a year after the knee injury, I began studying Kinetic Awareness with Elaine Summers in the hope that she could teach me how to overcome a long-standing problem I had with my upper back (a severe kyphosis). My posture was so bad that I could not go for more than an hour or so without lying down on my back to relieve the pain. I looked like a hunchback. Worse, my spine seemed immovable.

After two years with Elaine Summers, I had made substantial progress with my back (today it has recovered over 90%). At that time I asked her to look at my knee. After watching me do a few movements from the T'ai Chi Ch'uan form, she said, "You are putting enormous pressure on your knees, ankles, and arches." She then taught me the correct alignment.

For the next two weeks I assiduously practiced only two movements of the form: "Ward off Left" and "Ward off Right." I did these movements very slowly, scrupulously applying what she had just taught me about the alignment of my arches, ankles, and knees. At first, the new alignment felt totally alien and uncomfortable. When I mentioned this problem to her, she said, "Soon you will find that you are actually forcing your knees out of alignment. When you stop forcing, the correct alignment will occur without any effort." At the end of the two weeks of dedicated practice, my knee had recovered completely.

I explain my quick progress as follows: My knee had substantially recovered from the initial injury. However, without realizing it, I *had* been habitually forcing my knee into an incorrect alignment. The repeated stress on the injured ligament kept it from healing completely. Moreover, the pain that I was experiencing was necessary to warn me of a vulnerability. Because I had no idea of the correct alignment of the knee, it did not enter my mind that the pain and retarded healing stemmed from anything over which I had control. Once the vulnerability was eliminated by programming in proper use, the ligament could then fully heal. Then the pain was no longer required. The ligaments became secure because I was treating them with care.

Don Ahn, a T'ai Chi Ch'uan teacher in New York City, demonstrates the strength and stability that stem from correct alignment in the following way: He assumes a 70-30 posture and relaxes. He then asks someone to try to move his forward knee to the side. It is unmovable. This demonstration dramatically shows how stable the knee is when it is correctly aligned.

A Story About an Acquaintance

Recently, an acquaintance of mine was ice skating and fell. She sprained the fingers of one hand so badly that she could not use that hand for months. I wondered how she, an experienced ice skater, had managed to incur such an injury. I therefore became more observant of her movements.

I saw something that I remembered having noticed many times before her injury: She habitually placed not only her fingers but her wrists and elbows in precarious, extreme positions. It was evident to me that this habit led to her injury.

Alignment of the Hand and Wrist

Professor Cheng emphasized what he called the "beauteous hand," by which he meant the wrist and fingers when gently curved in a natural manner (see Fig. 5-1). The shape of the hand and wrist and the space between the fingers, affect the flow of ch'i to the hands to a surprising degree (also see the section on *Centering* in chapter

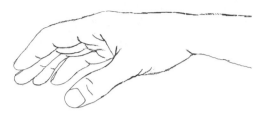

Fig. 5-1. *The "beauteous hand."*

2). Many practitioners whose lineage does not stem from Cheng Man-ch'ing finish movements with a bent wrist and a consequent focus into the heel of the hand. Other practitioners flex wrists during transitions in a manner that would occur if the wrist were extremely relaxed and the resistance of the air were many times greater than it actually is. In fact, it takes considerable tension to simulate the conditions suggested by both of these types of flexing. In defense of the flexing of the wrist in the final postures, some practitioners claim that they *would* use the palm heel in the case of an actual strike. This defense can be disputed for two reasons:

1. In an actual self-defense situation, the particular fist used is not formed until the moment of contact. In the case of a palm-heel strike, first the fingers would touch, and then the wrist would bend, allowing the palm heel to strike the opponent.

2. When dealing with the air it is unnecessary to introduce the level of tension corresponding to an actual strike. Rather, an important reason to practice without this tension is to sharpen sensitivity.

Some advanced practitioners make subtle shapes with their hands and flexing movements with their wrists in order to "squeeze" ch'i and thereby intensify it. I surmise that Professor Cheng discouraged us from doing such valid flexing because he had seen too many practitioners whose flexing movements involved only an outer appearance without any inner content.

Alignment of the Knees

The knee is a very vulnerable joint. It must support almost the full body weight. Because of the length of the leg bones, the resulting leverage can subject the knee joint to large stresses. For this reason, it is crucial to understand and incorporate the correct alignment of this joint. Before the alignment of the knee can be adequately discussed, it is necessary to introduce a useful term:

Definition: The axis of a bone is the straight line connecting the centers of the joints at both ends of that bone.

Even though a bone may have an irregular shape, its axis provides us with a straight line that is useful when discussing alignment. As we will see, joints have the least harmful stress placed upon them when force is directed along the axes of the bones instead of at an angle to those axes.

The knee joint is the intersection of two bones, the femur (thigh bone) and the tibia (shin bone) (see Fig. 5-2). The femur is quite irregular and has, near its uppermost end, a large protrusion called the greater trochanter. Many people who do not have an understanding of anatomy erroneously think that the *greater trochanter* is the thigh joint. They make this error because they think in terms of the outer shape of the bone. Once it is understood that the femur makes a sharp inward bend near the top, it is better to disregard the outer appearance of the bone and think in terms of the axis of the bone.

The following criterion applies to the proper alignment of the knee joint:

When all the weight of the body is on one leg, with the knee substantially bent (as is typical of many T'ai Chi Ch'uan stances and transitions), for zero harmful lateral stress, the knee must be directly above the center line of the foot (Fig. 5-3).

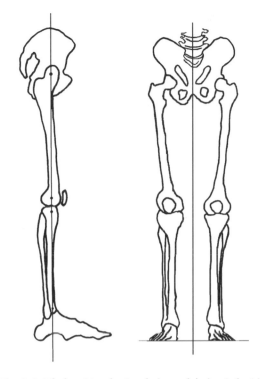

Fig. 5-2. *The knee joint showing the bones of the leg. Left: side view, right: front view.*

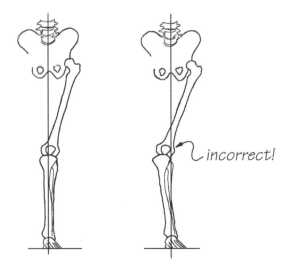

Fig. 5-3. *Correct (left) and incorrect (right) alignment of the knee joint.*

Since the center of mass of the body must be directly above the 100% weighted foot, the properly aligned knee joint then is in a state of compression with no lateral shearing force.

Many beginners of T'ai Chi Ch'uan—and even some advanced practitioners—habitually cave the knee inward from the ideal alignment just described. This habit places a harmful shearing stress on both the knee and ankle joints.

The knee is usually thought of as a "hinge joint" that bends with the axis of the femur always in the plane formed by the axis of the tibia and the center line of the foot. However, the following considerations will show that to eliminate shearing stress on the knee joint, the femur must move out of this plane: In a 100% stance, the center of mass of the body must be directly above the center line of the weighted foot. Also, for zero shear, the knee joint must be above the center line of the 100% weighted foot. Therefore, the center of mass, knee joint, and center line of the foot should all lie in the same vertical plane when 100% of the weight is on that leg. Thus it can be seen that when the leg is 100% weighted and in the proper alignment, the axis of the femur does not lie in the plane formed by the center line of the foot and the knee joint but is off to the side.

Alignment of the Ankle

When the center of the ankle joint is not directly above the center line of the foot, there is a shear on the ankle joint. Such a condition makes a sprained ankle more probable when there is a sudden additional force produced by an unexpected depression in the ground. Heels on shoes exacerbate this condition because of the increased leverage.

The alignment of the ankle depends on the alignment of the knee (just discussed) and the alignment of the foot (discussed next).

Alignment of the Arch of the Foot

Many people cave in their arches as though the arch were a weight-bearing part of the foot. In fact, the arch should make no contact with the ground. Once the arch caves in, the natural shock-absorbing quality of the foot is lost. Moreover, inordinate pressure is placed on the first metatarsal. This pressure can eventually damage the bone, leading to bunions. Last, when the arch caves in, the ankle joint and knee tend to be brought inward from center, thereby increasing the likelihood of a sprained ankle or knee.

Note: An exercise that should help you to achieve correct alignment of the knees, ankles, and arches is described in chapter 8 under "Exercises for Improving Balance."

About Parallel Feet

Professor Cheng frequently talked about the importance of parallel feet. He introduced this concept in "Step back to Repulse Monkey," for which he insisted that the two feet step backward on parallel lines that are one shoulder width apart.

He also emphasized that the feet should be parallel in the "Beginning" posture. He told us the anatomical reason: When the feet are toed out, the femurs force the lower part of the pelvis forward. Conversely, when the feet are toed in, the femurs force the lower part of the pelvis backward. When the feet are parallel, the pelvis is free of forces that rotate it forward or backward, and, therefore, the muscles that hold the pelvis can relax. Thus, when the feet are parallel, the femurs intersect the pelvis at such an angle that the pelvis "floats" in optimal alignment.

Professor Cheng also told us that toeing out the feet obstructs ch'i from entering the weilu gate in the sacral area.[1]

Alignment of the Pelvis

During all T'ai Chi Ch'uan movement, the pelvis should not deviate from the natural alignment that occurs when the feet are parallel with straight but loose knees. Even in a low 100% stance, the pelvis should be completely free and float in a natural manner.

Alignment of the Head

T'ai Chi Ch'uan students are commonly told to regard the head as if suspended above by a string. This admonishment means that (1) the head should not incline forward or to the side, (2) the neck should not be tense, and (3) the head should have a buoyant quality. All of these requirements can be attained if the head is first allowed to balance on the top vertebra of the spine (the atlas). To locate the atlas, place the tip of each index finger on each of the bony protrusions behind the ears called the mastoid processes. The atlas is now midway between the two finger tips.

The head should be lifted very slightly, so that some of the weight is taken off the atlas. When the optimal degree of lifting is achieved, the flow of ch'i is maximized.

Alignment of the Shoulders

There is no need to lift the shoulders in any movement of the T'ai Chi Ch'uan form. Lifting the shoulders corresponds to a state of tension that reduces the ability to react quickly and efficiently. When your shoulder is lifted during push-hands practice, your partner can easily use that defect to control you.

Alignment of the Elbows

Beginners tend to lift the elbows, and they are thus told to let the elbows droop. However, after gross tension in the elbows subsides, you should experiment with letting the elbows become somewhat buoyant. The optimal space between the elbows and the body is found by feeling the strongest flow of ch'i and its consequent supportive effect on the arms.

Alignment of the Spine

The spine is naturally curved, and no knowledgeable person would suggest that the spine should be made straight. The curves of the spine act to absorb shock. If the spine were straight, with the vertebra stacked one upon the other, each footstep would cause a jolt to the whole body. Instead, the curves flex, thereby absorbing each impact.

Unfortunately, many people have spines that are excessively curved. Women (more than men) frequently have an accentuated curve of the lower back. People who sit at desks for long periods of time tend to have an accentuated curve of the upper back. Defects in the shape of the spine fall into three main categories: *scoliosis,* which is a lateral curvature of the spine (usually at two compensating places); *kyphosis,* which is an excessive outward curvature of the thorasic region of the spine; and *lordosis,* which is an excessive outward curvature, usually of the lumbar region of the spine.

As an excessive curvature increases, it is more difficult to reverse. The muscles on the outside of the curve are subjected to excessive tension, and the muscles on the inside of the curve become foreshortened. The greater the curvature, the larger the force required by the muscles around the spine to counteract the leverage produced and reduce the excessive curve. Also, if the discs of the spine, which are cushions between the vertebrae, are squashed on one side for a long time, they tend not to spring back to their optimal supportive shape. Thus, the muscular action required of the outer muscles to reduce the curvature becomes increasingly difficult and more painful. A person whose spine is excessively curved finds it easier to give in to gravity than to correct the situation, and the curvature continually worsens.

However, an advanced curvature of the spine *can* be successfully reversed, as evidenced by my own case mentioned earlier in this chapter.

Proper Sitting

When a child sits on the floor, not only are the leg muscles beneficially lengthened, but correct posture of the upper body is also learned. Children will spontaneously attain a squatting posture or sit on the floor on their heels, between their heels, or cross-legged. It is only when children are forced to wear shoes with hard backs, that these sitting positions become either corrupted or inhibited. For example, hard shoes make it difficult for children to sit on or between their heels with the feet pointed to the rear, as is physiologically optimal.

When children wearing hard shoes sit between their heels they point their feet outward to avoid the pressure of the back of the shoe on the Achilles tendon. The consequent twisting of the ankles and knees can cause later postural problems leading to sprains of these joints. Next, children who regularly slouch in soft chairs with backs are deprived of the necessity to learn correct posture. When children sit on the floor or on benches with no backs, they quickly attain an optimal posture of the spine. This posture becomes habitual. It is of interest that most skeletons used in anatomy classrooms, etc., come from Asians. Skeletons from Americans and Europeans so frequently have severe malformations of the spine that they are seldom used.

Note

1. See Cheng Man-ch'ing, *Cheng Tzu's Thirteen Treatises on T'ai Chi Ch'uan,* p. 150.

CHAPTER 6

Warm-Up and Stretching

Some T'ai Chi Ch'uan practitioners feel that preliminary warm-up and stretching are superfluous. However, warm-up and stretching are of great value to the practitioner and are crucial when doing other more vigorous forms of exercise or movement. A period of proper warm-up and stretching relaxes the body, quiets the mind, and, if repeated regularly, greatly increases overall flexibility. Moreover, there are many other benefits, which shall be discussed.

The concepts of this chapter were taught to me by Don Oscar Becque and Elaine Summers. Over the years I have observed, in both myself and my students, the value of what I learned from these teachers.

FLEXIBILITY

Whenever possible, observe people of all ages, and notice what characterizes the movements of young and old people. See if the major difference is that of flexibility. We are all born with essentially the full range of flexibility. All infants suck their big toes as easily as their thumbs. However, many elderly people have difficulty in moving through even a small fraction of the range accessible to an infant.

Why Do We Lose Flexibility?

It is a mistake to think that loss of flexibility is a necessary part of the aging process. The truth is that flexibility decreases with the number of
years that the body is deprived of its full range of movement. The aging process in this regard is not related to the age of the individual but to the number of years spent in wrong or incomplete use.

Why is Flexibility Important?

There are three basic reasons why flexibility is important:

1. Flexibility determines the extent to which the body can adjust to conditions of vulnerability. The larger the range of motion, the greater the options of adaptation. To the extent that movement is limited, so are options for adaptation.

2. Every movement we make facilitates the flow of lymph and serves to massage, nourish, cleanse, and oxygenate the muscles, organs, glands, blood vessels, nerves, and channels of ch'i known as meridians. In addition, every movement strengthens bones and cartilage. To the extent that flexibility is reduced, these benefits are correspondingly reduced.

3. Flexibility of the body and the mind go hand in hand. The loss or gain of bodily flexibility cannot occur without a corresponding loss or gain of mental flexibility.

WARM-UP

Before any demanding movement is undertaken, it is important to do a "warm-up" by gently moving all of the joints of the body throughout their range. This movement allows the synovial fluid of the joints to become distributed and is a perfect way of initiating the toning and oxygenating process of stretching. A warm-up involves rotation and/or flexing of the joints of the fingers, wrists, elbows, shoulders, jaw, spine, pelvis, knees, ankles, and toes. Additionally, muscles of the face, eyes, and breathing apparatus should be gently activated.

It is a mistake to think that a warm-up can be achieved by vigorous calisthenics such as push-ups, jumping jacks, and rapid toe touching. Such activities should be undertaken only after a true warm-up, if at all.

STRETCHING

Stretching is a spontaneous activity that can be observed in all animals and even in insects. Unfortunately, to a great extent, human beings have lost the innate urge to stretch. This loss is largely because of societal pre-programming. When we were children, most of us were discouraged by parents and teachers from engaging in movements that would draw attention to ourselves or lessen our effectiveness in the machine-age, work-a-day, assembly-line world in which we live and must function. At an early age, children are customarily weaned of moving in accordance with inner impulses and are trained to eventually spend a full eight-hour day at a desk or machine. Of course, self-discipline and control of our impulses are valuable, if not essential. However, in completely subduing these natural impulses, we incur a heavy price.

These days, many young children are less flexible than some middle-aged adults who properly use their bodies. Studies show that the average child spends more time sitting in front of a television set than in any other activity. To make things worse, in schools, children are not encouraged to sit on the floor, as is the custom in Asian cultures but, instead, on ill-designed chairs with backs. This practice leads to slouching.

The Benefits of Stretching

Many people think that the only benefit of stretching is an increase in flexibility. When increased flexibility is not observed, discouragement sets in. However, stretching has many benefits beyond that of flexibility. Stretching beneficially stresses the bones, which prevents them from releasing calcium and becoming weak and brittle. Moreover, stretching tones the muscles, organs, glands, blood vessels, nerves, and channels of ch'i. Cats sleep as much as fourteen hours per day and engage in little physical activity other than frequent stretching, but they remain in top physical condition and are always ready to spring into action.

During stretching of the kind in which the mind is keenly attuned to inner natural processes such as breathing, tension of muscles, etc., the mind is discovering and experiencing directly rather than comparing or characterizing. Emotions, expectations, and preconceptions are subdued. Thus stretching conduces to a meditative state.

The Importance of Stretching Correctly

A recent awareness of the importance of flexibility and other health-related factors has inspired many people to incorporate stretching into a daily exercise program. Exercise is a way of making up for a manner of living that does not involve the right kind or the right amount of movement and expenditure of physical energy. Because exercise is contrived and is done by many people without an internal dialogue between the mind and the tissues, there is a high potential for harm. Moreover, our idea of what is best for us often does not stem from a correct understanding of physiology. To make things worse, we tend to expect immediate results.

In exercise we are consciously or unconsciously programming into our minds and bodies the way in which we will later move as reflex. Therefore, it is essential that we program the correct ideas. If, in the name of exercise, we abuse our bodies, aside from doing immediate harm, this abusive manner of moving will also pervade other movements. Programming a way of moving that subjects our tissues to vulnerability will ultimately lead to injury and harm. Conversely, proper stretching re-educates our bodies to move more healthfully, more economically, and with less vulnerability.

There are a number of pitfalls and incorrect ideas about stretching. For example, to most people, the word *stretch* implies exerting a force on both ends of something in an attempt to make it longer, as in the case of stretching a rubber band. This interpretation of *stretching* is responsible for much harm. In fact, the most beneficial effects of stretching occur when the muscles extend *voluntarily* rather than being mercilessly overpowered by a stronger set of opposing muscles and leverage. For example, when most people are asked to touch their toes, they will bend over, pull forward, and jam their knees back, contracting the muscles in the front of the body in order to elongate the muscles on the back of the legs (hamstrings). This method of stretching is exactly the opposite of what would be most beneficial.

To learn the best way to stretch, watch a cat. They stretch following an *inner feeling* rather than an *idea* of how their body should move. Cats perform their version of a forward stretch by lifting their coccyx and *extending* their hamstrings. To illustrate the distinction to my students, I use the following analogy:

Consider an open book held as shown in Fig. 6-1. Let the uppermost edges of the pages, which are held from above, represent the hip joint, and let the spine of the book represent the knee. The lowermost edges of the pages represent the foot.

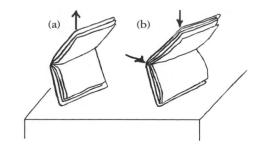

Fig. 6-1. *(a) Correct and (b) incorrect ways of stretching, as illustrated by opening a book two ways. The arrows show the direction of applied forces.*

One way that the book can open further is to lift the part held with the hand (Fig. 6-1a). This corresponds to the knee moving passively as a result of the muscles in the back of the legs elongating on their own and is correct.

The other way to open the book further is to push back its spine (Fig. 6-1b). This way corresponds to jamming back the knee by tensing the muscles in the front part of the leg, causing the muscles in the back of the legs to be elongated. Of course, jamming the knee back is not the correct way of stretching the hamstrings.

Ideally, the muscles involved become longer by extending voluntarily instead of being forced to elongate by a stronger set of opposing muscles with the use of leverage.

There is an analogy between proper stretching and a meeting of people who are devoted to arriving at a consensus. Ideally, the goal should be for the people involved not to take a course of action until those who disagree are genuinely convinced by the others. Similarly, in stretching, no action should be taken unless all muscle fibers can participate painlessly. If there is any fiber that cannot comfortably go along with the action, the limiting fiber should not be forced by the others. Instead, the action should be suspended while that fiber is assisted by the mind in releasing its resistance to lengthening.

Monitoring Progress

Because the process of recovering flexibility and range is relatively slow, it is easy to become discouraged. When we get an immediate result or see progress, it inspires us to continue, but when progress is of such a nature that it is invisible, we tend to become discouraged. Discouragement leads to an unnatural forcing or to giving up too quickly.

When there is a large distance to go, a given increase in flexibility is much less noticeable than when the distance is small. Also, the less flexible you are, the more your muscles will tend to protest against the stretching that they need. Thus, the more you need to do stretching, the more important it is *not* to monitor progress but to feel the internal benefits to the organs, the flow of ch'i, and the improvement of muscle tone. Keep in mind the other important benefits of stretching beyond that of merely increasing flexibility.

Arresting or Reversing Inflexibility

People of all ages can increase their flexibility and get many other additional benefits through proper stretching. There are three levels of progress. At the first level, flexibility continues to decrease but at a lower rate than if stretching were not done. At the next level, the same degree of flexibility is maintained. At the third level, flexibility increases. With daily correct stretching, the third level can be attained by people of all ages.

Experiencing the Effect of Each Action

In any form of bodily activity, it is essential to experience the effects of each action. The more the mind is involved, the greater the benefit. Each stretch has an effect on the mind, muscles, organs, circulation of blood, circulation of ch'i, etc. Following these effects with the mind intensifies them. With time, a minimum of physical action will be required to achieve a given effect. Eventually, that effect can be accomplished by the mind alone.

Further, by resting after a stretching movement and experiencing the effect, you can learn about the state of the body and the degree to which each feature of the movement improved that state. This way, the best manner of stretching will be learned first hand. Also, when you fully experience the benefit of an action, future repetition of that action requires less will power. Motivation will naturally stem from sensing the needs of the tissues and from an awareness that a particular action will satisfy those needs.

Getting Up After Stretching

After a period of meditative stretching on the floor, it is especially important to rise to a standing position *slowly*. There are three reasons for adopting this practice:

1. During meditation or periods of quiet, the circulatory system rests and slows down. Getting up too fast puts a sudden strain on a quiescent circulatory system and should be avoided.

2. During stretching, muscles are coaxed into an unaccustomed range of motion. Muscles can be harmed if they are suddenly forced to tense while in this vulnerable state. Moreover, the muscles will be much less likely to allow themselves to be subjected to such vulnerability in the future, and progress will be reduced.

   For example, lying on your back for a period of time lengthens the muscles on the inside of the spine in the region of the upper back. These muscles are exactly the ones that are required to tense when the upper body is lifted, as occurs in a sit-up. Instead of rising head first, it is better to roll over slowly onto one side and rest for a while. Then, using the forearm on that side, slowly come up to sitting on your heels. After sitting for a short period, come up to your knees, put one foot forward, and slowly come up to standing.

3. One of the most important benefits of stretching is the releasing of prior patterns and fixations of tension. It is of great benefit to come to standing from a prone position without jumping back to the old patterns.

The Best Time of Day to Stretch

Some people believe that stretching in the early morning is the best. Others believe that it is better to wait until later in the day, when the muscles are less stiff. While it is true that *incorrect* stretching does more harm to stiff muscles than to loose muscles, *correct* stretching sensitively takes into account the limitations, vulnerabilities, and needs of stiff muscles. The stiffer the muscles are, the more important it is that correct stretching be done and done promptly. From my experience, stretching in the early morning results in obtaining benefits earlier in the day and a greater range of movement throughout the day.

A possible reason that muscles are stiff after a night's sleep is that during sleep there is a lack of activity of the lymph system and kidneys. This inactivity results in muscles becoming waterlogged and therefore stiff.

Yawning

Earlier, it was stated that we have lost the innate urge to stretch. However, there is one that remains: *the yawn.* A yawn is the extension of the muscles of the respiratory tract. There is a widespread misconception that yawning results from the body's general need for more oxygen. If this idea were true, yawning would be *less,* not *more* frequent after doing deep breathing. However, the reverse is true: The more one breathes, the more one yawns. Notice that when you yawn, the action is more for the stretching of the muscles of respiration than for a general intake of oxygen.

If we become aware of what happens during a yawn, we will learn the feeling of correct stretching.

Spontaneous Stretching

Once the pain associated with out-of-tone muscles eventually subsides, it is possible to experience the spontaneous desire of muscles to extend. There must first be a period of listening to the needs of the muscles and allowing them to do what they want rather than bossing them around with our idea of what we think they need. Then, even during sleep, subtle or overt stretching will become spontaneous.

Stretching Using Gravity

After the muscles have been moved throughout their range by extending them (instead of subjecting them to a pull at each end by opposing muscles) it is permissible to use gravity in the stretching process. While the effect of gravity does provide a pull at both ends, gravity is predictable and dependable. Moreover, gravity is external and makes it easy to relax and submit to its pull. The following will illustrate how gravity can be used.

Hanging

Stand with the feet parallel and somewhat less than a shoulder width apart. More precisely, the center of each ankle joint should be directly below the center of each corresponding thigh joint (see Fig. 5-2). Keeping the legs straight but the knees loose, let the top of the body bend forward to a hanging position. Then shift the weight forward without clenching the toes. Allow the head and shoulders to droop. For some people, the hands will be quite above the feet, but, with time, the palm heels should eventually touch the floor. The entire body should give in to gravity, and the mind should work on releasing that which is restricted.

The least stressful way of getting up from a hanging position is to bend your knees and lower your coccyx as the trunk of your body moves into a vertical orientation. Then come up to standing by straightening your legs. This manner of rising reduces the stress on the vertebrae of the lower back.

Hanging requires the circulatory system to pump blood against gravity, whereas, previously, there was a "free ride." Thus, a fringe benefit of hanging is the exercise of some of the arterial muscles that would otherwise tend to atrophy.

Stretching Using Momentum

It is permissible to use momentum only after the muscles have become fully toned by first extending them and then stretching using gravity. For example, after spending some time hanging, you can lift your upper body and then release it so that it drops down with a bounce. With repetition, the bouncing can become higher and higher, so that the entire upper body raises and lowers at a "resonant frequency." The springiness and inertia of the body will determine a natural rate at which the motion will build. This motion is similar to that of a child on a swing when given optimally timed pushes.

Be aware that momentum reduces sensitivity and control and, therefore, has potential to do harm. Unfortunately, many people disregard both warming up and thorough initial stretching. Instead, they immediately proceed to strenuous movements using momentum. Such a manner of treating the body is the opposite of self-improvement.

The Importance of Stretching Equally in Both Directions

For every forward stretch there should be a corresponding backward stretch, and, for every stretch to one side, there should be another to the opposite side. This alternation ensures that each set of muscles gets equal benefit.

The Importance of Repeating Each Stretch

It is a good idea to repeat both sides or directions of each stretch. Aside from the fact that more stretching is accomplished, repetition gives an immediate opportunity to assess the improvement achieved by each action.

"Cracking" of Joints

During movement, a cracking sound is occasionally heard coming from various joints. Is this cracking good or bad? Some say that frequent cracking of joints causes arthritis. While severe stress to joints is a cause of arthritis and is to be avoided, the natural cracking of joints is quite beneficial.

The following is my explanation of why one type of cracking occurs. When joints are not moved for a period of time, the two adjacent layers of cartilage become compressed and slightly flattened. At the same time, the increased area of contact causes the synovial fluid, which ordinarily separates and lubricates the surfaces of the cartilage, to be squeezed out. When the joint is then moved, instead of the surfaces gliding as they should, they roll without slipping. This rolling tends to open up one side of the joint, placing the ligaments of that side of the joint under tension. When the tension is enough to overcome the friction of the cartilaginous surfaces, the joint breaks free and moves for a short distance. The joint settles into place with a snap. An analogous situation is a kitchen table whose legs have settled into the linoleum floor over a period of time. When the table is moved, a certain force has to build up before the legs break loose from the floor.

The cracking of joints sets up a beneficial vibration in the bones and ligaments and allows the synovial fluid to be distributed throughout the joint. Further, the consequent release of muscular tension and blockages of ch'i are highly beneficial. Chiropractic recognizes the benefit of cracking joints.

It should be noted that the above cracking of joints cannot be immediately repeated because the cracking eliminates its cause. Cracking that can immediately be repeated is not a good sign. This cracking can be caused by muscles that are so contracted that they repeatedly pull a joint out of alignment each time a particular movement occurs, causing the bones to jump. Here, it is best to work around *this* cracking by choosing a slightly different path of movement.

Caution: Cracking of a joint using any force that *jams* the joint together is to be avoided. Instead, there should be a gentle force that *separates* the bones.

CHAPTER 7

Stances

The stances (final postures) of T'ai Chi Ch'uan are designed to provide an optimal combination of stability, safety, and mobility. Descriptive terms will first be defined to help the practitioner understand and refer to the precise details of the basic stances.

DEFINITIONS OF TERMS

Planes and Lines

Medial Plane of the Body. A vertical plane through the midline of the body that divides the body into right and left halves (see Fig. 7-1).

Frontal Plane. A vertical plane at right angles to the medial plane, dividing the body into anterior and posterior portions (see Fig. 7-1).

Medial Plane of the Head. A vertical plane through the midline of the head that divides the head into right and left halves. (When the nose and navel line up, the medial planes of the body and head are coincident.)

Center Line of a Foot. A line on the sole of the foot from the center of the sole at its widest part to the center of the heel (see Fig. 7-2).

Terms Describing Stances

Each stance has six main attributes: *width, length, weight distribution, spatial direction, angle of the rear foot,* and *integrity.*

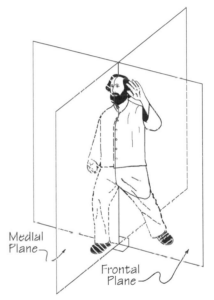

Fig. 7-1. *The planes of the body.*

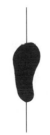

Fig. 7-2. *The center line of the foot.*

Width. The (perpendicular) distance W from the heel of the rear foot to the center line of the forward foot (see Fig. 7-3).

Length. The distance L from the heel of the rear foot to the heel of the forward foot, as measured along the center line of the forward foot (see Fig. 7-3).

Weight Distribution. The relative portion of body weight borne by each foot. (In a 70-30 stance, the forward foot bears 70% of the weight, and the rear foot bears 30%.)

Direction. The direction of a stance is usually taken to be the forward direction of the center line of the forward foot (see Fig. 7-3). In some stances the medial plane of the body is not parallel to the direction of the stance. However, in all stances the

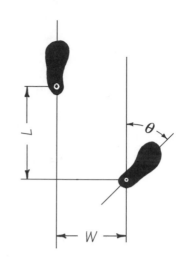

Fig. 7-3. *Terms describing stances, as illustrated in the 70-30 stance.*

medial plane of the head is always parallel to the direction of the stance. Directions are commonly specified by the cardinal points of the compass: N, E, S, and W and the diagonal directions: NE, SE, SW, and NW. In this book, the form is arbitrarily assumed to begin with the practitioner facing north.

Angle of Rear Foot. The angle θ that the center line of the foot makes with the direction of the forward foot (see Fig. 7-3).

Integrity. The correct relative positions or orientations of the different body parts such as the pelvis, feet, knees, and head.

Additional Terms

Feet-Parallel. A condition that applies when the center lines of the feet are parallel.

Shoulder Width. The spacing of the centers of the shoulder joints. When you stand with your feet parallel and a shoulder width apart, the distance between the center lines of your feet is equal to the distance between the centers of your shoulder joints. An approximate shoulder width is achieved by making the spacing of the outsides of the shoulders equal to that of the outsides of the feet.

Double Weighting. A defect that occurs when orientation of your body is such that the reaction (in the sense of Newton's third law) to a force that you apply in the forward direction easily unbalances your body.

Square. A condition that applies when, in a stance, the frontal plane is perpendicular to the center line of the forward foot.

Empty. A condition that applies to a foot that exerts no pressure on the floor even if it touches it. Emptiness of a foot can be tested by placing a sheet of tissue paper on the floor under that foot. Then have another person try to remove the paper without tearing it. The foot is empty only if the paper can be removed intact.

DESCRIPTIONS OF THE MAIN STANCES
Fifty-Fifty Stance With Straight Knees

This stance occurs at the beginning and end of the form as taught by Cheng Man-ch'ing. In this stance, the feet are parallel, a shoulder width apart, and equally weighted.

It is considered a fault to assume a stationary posture in which the weight is evenly divided between two feet (fault of "double weighting"). However, the 50-50 stance has value as a meditative or Ch'i Kung posture.

Integrity of the 50-50 Stance. The knees in the 50-50 stance should be "straight but loose." To make this concept precise, consider the axes of the leg bones. (The axis of a bone is a line that begins at the center of the joint at one extreme of the bone and ends at the center of the joint at the other extreme.) The axes of the upper and lower leg bones should be collinear and lie in the frontal plane.

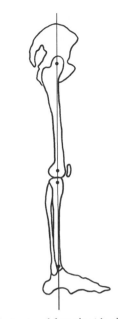

Fig. 7-4. *As viewed from the side, the axes of the leg bones are vertical and collinear in the 50-50 stance with straight knees.*

Moreover, the center of mass of the body is likewise in this plane (see Fig. 7-4).

Test: "Shadow movements" (minute movements for testing for centering) of the knees should be tried. Additionally, forward and backward movements of the whole body pivoting at the ankle joints are useful. When the correct alignment is achieved, it is possible to relax the muscles in the legs while standing in equilibrium. Only minor tensing is occasionally required to readjust the balance.

The leg muscles are very strong and do not easily release their accustomed tension. Therefore it may be a while before the 50-50 stance with straight knees is achieved. Once you master it, you can stand for long periods of time, luxuriating in the feeling that results from relaxed feet and legs.

Meditative Fifty-Fifty Stance

Another 50-50 stance suitable for long periods of meditative standing[1] is as follows: Instead of placing the feet a shoulder width apart, place the center of each ankle joint directly below the center of each corresponding thigh joint (see Fig. 7-5). Since the separation of the centers of the thigh joints is less than that of the shoulder joints, the width of this stance is less than a shoulder width. The axes of the leg bones are still in the frontal plane but now are vertical as viewed from the front.

As viewed from the front, in the meditative 50-50 stance, each thigh joint is located approximately midway between the center line of the body and the outside of the hip, just above the level of the pubic bone (see Fig. 7-6). As viewed from the side, the thigh joints are approximately midway between the front and rear of the body (see Fig. 7-7). Because the thigh joints are so deeply embedded in the pelvis, they are very difficult to locate by feel.

Fifty-Fifty Stance with Bent Knees

T'ai Chi Ch'uan practitioners who do not trace their lineage to Cheng Man-ch'ing do the "Beginning" posture in the 50-50 stance with bent knees, and there is certainly no objection to this traditional method. However, Cheng wanted us to experience the highly valuable state of relaxation that occurs in the 50-50 stance with straight knees. Since all other postures in the T'ai Chi Ch'uan form afford an opportunity to experience the strengthening benefits of bent knees, Cheng's modification seems to sacrifice little.

Seventy-Thirty Stance

This stance is so termed because 70% of the weight is on the forward foot and 30% is on the rear foot (see Fig. 7-3). It is more of a *final striking* or *pushing* stance than a *waiting* or *defensive* stance. It is used extensively in push-hands. The 70-30 stance occurs in both the cardinal and diagonal directions.

Width of the 70-30 Stance. The width of the 70-30 stance is a shoulder width. If the 70-30 stance is too narrow, the ability to turn both the body and the rear foot is restricted. Moreover, lateral balance is reduced. If the 70-30 stance is too wide, turning is again restricted, and forward and backward mobility is limited. For this reason, any alteration of the 70-30 stance can only be in the length—not the width, which must always be a shoulder width.

Test: To test a 70-30 stance for proper width, rotate the rear foot on its heel until it is parallel to the front foot. The center lines of both feet should now be a shoulder width apart.

Length of the 70-30 Stance. Ideally, the length of the 70-30 stance is such that the distance (in the direction of the forward foot)

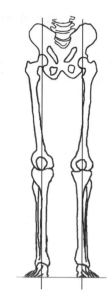

Fig. 7-5. As *viewed from the front, the axes of the leg bones are vertical and collinear in the meditative 50-50 stance.*

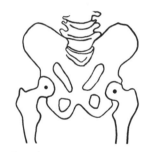

Fig. 7-6. A *front view of the pelvis, showing the location of the thigh joints.*

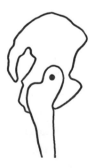

Fig. 7-7. A *side view of the pelvis showing the location of the thigh joints.*

from the heel of the forward foot to the ball of the rear foot is also a shoulder width (see Fig. 7-3). If you cannot legitimately attain a stance of this length, you should step into the greatest possible length without prematurely committing your weight or compromising width.

Tests: To test your optimal stance length (different for each person), stand with 100% of your weight on your rear leg, with your rear foot at 45°. Sink *totally* into the rear foot. Place the other foot as far forward as possible, maintaining a shoulder width and keeping the forward foot empty. Now the empty foot is positioned at the maximum length it can legally attain in a 70-30 stance.

If the forward foot of a 70-30 stance is too far forward (stance too long), then, when the weight is shifted back completely to the rear foot, the forward foot will slide backwards along the floor. This slippage implies that the previous step into this stance was one that improperly committed the weight. If the forward foot of a 70-30 stance is not sufficiently far forward (stance too short), the forward knee will be too bent when the weight is shifted back 100% to the rear foot. These tests can be used to determine the optimal length of each individual's 70-30 stance.

Integrity of the 70-30 Stance. The medial planes of both the body and head should be parallel to the center line of the forward foot. Alternatively stated, the nose and navel both should point in the same direction as that of the forward foot.

When the navel points at an angle with the direction of the forward foot, or, equivalently, when the forward foot is angled outward, that foot is easily "swept" by the opponent. Conversely, when the forward foot is pointed forward or is angled inward, the forward foot tends to wedge into the floor and makes it harder to be swept.

The knee of the rear leg is substantially bent.[2] The rear foot is flat on the floor, instead of collapsing inward onto the arch and first metatarsal. Therefore the ankle of the rear foot is substantially bent.

The maximum extension of the forward knee occurs when a plumb line dropped from the kneecap passes through the ball of the big toe of the forward foot (see Fig. 7-8).

Tests: It is necessary to position the eyes *directly above* the knee when testing to see that the knee does not extend past the toe. When you look at your knee with your head in its proper alignment for the stance, the knee seems to be more forward than it actually is.

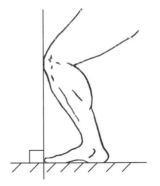

Fig. 7-8. *The maximum extension of the forward knee in a 70-30 stance.*

This optical illusion is caused by the fact that the eyes are not directly above the knee but behind it.

Here is an another way of calibrating the positioning of the forward knee: Touch the toe of the forward foot to a wall. Then assume a 70-30 stance. Bring the knee forward until it also touches the wall. Then carefully note the feeling and appearance so that they will be remembered later.

The weight distribution may be checked by using a scale. First weigh yourself. Then assume a 70-30 stance with the forward foot on the scale and the rear foot on an object of the same height as the scale. The scale reading should be your weight multiplied by 0.70.

Often students find it difficult to get appreciable weight onto the forward foot without over-extending in the forward direction. The way to overcome this problem is to shift the center of mass of the body laterally in the direction that loads the forward foot. For example, in shifting into a 70-30 stance with the left foot forward, it is necessary to shift the center of mass of the body to the left as well as forward.

Angle of the Rear Foot. The rear foot makes an angle of 45° with the forward direction. Failure to achieve 45° frequently results from not linking the rear leg with the body during turning.

Diagonal Seventy-Thirty Stance

This stance is exactly the same as the normal 70-30 stance just discussed except that the direction of this stance is diagonal.

In the diagonal 70-30 stance in, say, the NE direction, as in "Diagonal Flying," the forward foot points NE and the rear foot points N. Furthermore, the heel of the forward foot is on a line that (a) is perpendicular to the center line of the rear foot and (b) intersects that foot at a point midway between its heel and ball (see Fig. 7-9).

Even though the relative orientation of the feet in the diagonal 70-30 stance is the same as that for the ordinary 70-30 stance, the diagonal version is difficult for beginners to achieve. Stepping into the diagonal 70-30 stance from a cardinal direction is difficult for two reasons: (1) It requires strength, balance, and openness of the thigh joints (a full 135°) to take the required step, and (2) the diagonal direction is disorienting. Consequently, there is a tendency to lose the correct width and integrity of the final posture. Those who have difficulty in stepping into a diagonal 70-30 stance are advised to check that the stationary foot is in the correct position to begin with and that the stepping

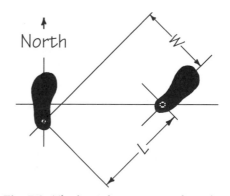

Fig. 7-9. *The diagonal 70-30 stance shown for a stance facing in the NE direction.*

foot does not angle out. Then, as a last resort, reduce the angle of the diagonal 70-30 stance from 135°. For example, instead of stepping 135° to the NE, you might step only $90°+22.5°=112.5°$ to ENE. However, no modification can occur at the expense of the width of the stance, which is sacred.

One-Hundred-Percent Stance.

In the 100% stance, all the weight is on the rear foot, with the forward foot empty.

Integrity. The rear foot makes an angle of 45° (sometimes 90°) with respect to the forward foot. The center line of the forward foot passes through the heel of the rear foot. The medial plane of the body is at about 45° to the forward direction. The knee of the weighted foot is above the center line of that foot—not buckled laterally inward. Because the center of gravity of the body is directly over the center line of the weighted foot, the hip on the weighted side appears to protrude to that side.

A Note of Caution

The kneecap of the 100% leg should be above the center line of the corresponding foot (see Fig. 7-10). If the knee caves inward from this position, there is a shearing stress on the ligaments of that knee, and that knee (and ankle) is vulnerable to being sprained. An injury might not occur while practicing T'ai Chi Ch'uan, but, because of the incorrect practice, the wrong alignment will be habituated into the movements of everyday life. An injury is more likely to occur in a hazardous or awkward situation such as inadvertently stepping off an unseen curb.

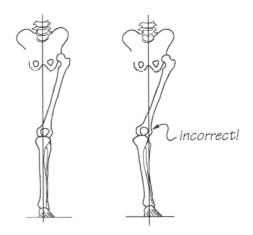

In certain 100% postures, it is both possible and beneficial to increase the angle from 45° to as much as 90° but only if the hip joint can open without the weighted knee buckling in, as just described.

Fig. 7-10. *The correct and incorrect alignment of the weighted knee in a 100% stance.*

There are two versions of 100% stances: One version is with the ball or the heel of the forward foot touching the floor but exerting no pressure on the floor. The other is with the forward foot raised. It is more difficult to maintain balance with the foot raised, since there is a lack of sense data that otherwise would be provided by the contact of the foot with the floor.

The 100% stance is a ready, fighting stance. First, it protects against being swept by the opponent because no weight is committed to the forward foot.

Second, the forward foot is ready to kick, step, or deflect a kick without any preliminary transfer of weight. Such a transfer would "telegraph" one's intention to the opponent.

In a 100% stance the navel points at about 45° to the direction of the stance. At this angle, the body presents less of a target than if the body were square to the stance. However, the nose always points in the direction of the stance.

Note that in the 100% stance the weighted knee is permitted to extend *beyond* the toe.

Notes

1. It should be noted that a standing posture is ideal for doing meditation. The bones of the lower body are much more suited for locomotion or standing than for sitting.

2. Many Yang-style practitioners *do not* bend the rear knee. For a discussion, see chapter 10, under "Variations in Interpretation of the T'ai Chi Ch'uan Movements."

CHAPTER 8

On Being a Student

When people ask you how long you have studied T'ai Chi Ch'uan, don't tell them the number of years; tell them the number of hours of practice logged.

—William C. C. Chen

One of the most important dividends gained from the study of T'ai Chi Ch'uan is an approach to learning. An approach to learning is much more valuable than any subject matter because it can be applied to *any* subject matter. For this reason, for thousands of years, the Chinese and neighboring cultures have emphasized process rather than results.

This chapter contains venerable methods, concepts, and attitudes that were inculcated in me by the T'ai Chi Ch'uan and spiritual masters under whom I have studied.

T'AI CHI CH'UAN PRACTICE

The Importance of Practice

My first teacher, Cheng Man-ch'ing, said that there are three factors that determine the rate at which the student learns and benefits from T'ai Chi Ch'uan: (1) correct teaching, (2) natural talent, and (3) perseverance (practice). Of the three, natural ability is the least important, and correct teaching or right method is the most important.[1]

Once a teacher has been selected, correct teaching is not in the hands of the student. Natural ability is also a given. Thus, the only factor over which a student has full and continuing control is practice.

There are two main aspects of practice. One aspect is that consistent practice increases the benefits of T'ai Chi Ch'uan. Some of these benefits are improved balance, coordination, and reflexes; calmness of mind; patience; concentration; self-awareness; and stronger bones, muscles, and organs. The other aspect is that correct practice involves continued learning and new insights, which, over a period of time, greatly increase the richness of the benefits achieved.

Class is Not Practice

It is essential that the student realize that going to class does not substitute for individual practice. Attending class without practicing on your own is analogous to taking a math course, copying down the problems done at the board by the teacher, and failing to do homework. The purpose of class is mainly for the presentation of new material. It is up to the student to absorb and incorporate that material through diligent and thorough independent practice. There must be the proper balance of self-initiated study with the structured presentations and activities in class.

Continuity of Practice.

In the words of Benjamin Pang Jeng Lo, "T'ai Chi Ch'uan has no vacations." There are a number of reasons never to miss a day of T'ai Chi Ch'uan practice. One reason is that there is a certain continuity necessary for progress. If a day is missed, there is a strong possibility that the mind will irrevocably lose the thread of both that learned in class and that being worked on. When an insight or breakthrough is ready to occur, it is important that the vehicle for its actualization be available. In T'ai Chi Ch'uan there is no "final result." Rather, there is a gradual accumulation of benefits that compound like savings in a high-interest account. Therefore, a small set-back at the beginning substantially reduces future accumulations.

When I was working on my doctoral dissertation in experimental physics, a co-worker said, "Every day's work you miss is one day later that you will get your Ph.D." However, I became aware that missing a day had an even greater negative effect. Missing a day made the next day harder and less efficient. When I was active, a certain momentum began to build. When I was inactive, a corresponding inertia prevailed and became increasingly difficult to overcome.

Another reason not to miss a day's practice is that if one day is missed, another can just as easily be missed, and so on. I make it a rule never to retire without having practiced that day. Cheng Man-ch'ing used to say, "Ten minutes of T'ai Chi Ch'uan is better than ten minutes more sleep." At the end of a day when I think that I am too tired to do the form, I remember Cheng's words. After ten minutes of practice, I am frequently so energized that I end up practicing much more than ten minutes. When I finally go to bed, my sleep is much deeper and better than if I had not practiced. The next day I experience an increased efficiency. Moreover, daily practice over a period of time results in a lowering of the need for sleep by much more than the time spent practicing.

Still another reason for not missing practice is that a certain rate of progress is expected by the teacher. If insufficient progress is evident, the teacher tends to expend less energy in teaching that student. It is somewhat disappointing for a teacher to correct a student and next class see no evidence that the correction has been worked on. (The absence of any verbal reference on the teacher's part to the student's progress does not mean that the teacher does not observe that progress or its lack.)

The student who fails to practice this difficult art regularly will have a dual sense of failure (1) from a lack of self-discipline and (2) from a lack of progress. The student will unconsciously say, "I am not good at T'ai Chi Ch'uan" and will feel that T'ai Chi Ch'uan is not as good as it is claimed to be. This notion will give both the student and T'ai Chi Ch'uan a bad name in the student's own mind.

Group or Individual Practice?

Group practice has many benefits. One benefit is that the combined energy and enthusiasm of the group augments that of each individual. Usually ch'i is experienced more intensely when practicing in a group. Another benefit is that group practice widens an awareness of spatial relations, timing, and intentions of others. Moreover, a major benefit of group practice is that students can observe others' movements and, by noticing differences, become aware of their own deficiencies. When you do T'ai Chi Ch'uan alone, your mind coordinates all of your body parts harmoniously. When you practice in a group, your mind now processes the movement, timing, and spacing of other people in the group. This processing adds a further dimension of harmony and connectedness.

In China, group practice of T'ai Chi Ch'uan is common. However, a close look at (or a photograph of) such a group will probably reveal that some of these practitioners have their heads turned so that they can copy the leader. They can only do T'ai Chi Ch'uan in a group. They need to watch the leaders constantly to know what movement comes next. It is unlikely that much of the meditative benefits can accrue when the student does not even know the movements by heart.

There are certain important benefits of individual practice that cannot be obtained from group practice:

1. When you practice independently, you can stop and repeat a movement or sequence of movements. Moreover, you can attain the optimal speed (discussed later in this chapter under "Ways of Practicing").

2. Practicing independently develops self-reliance and self-discipline. When you cannot copy others' movements or ask them questions, you must work things out alone. When there is not a practice time set by others, more self-motivation is required.

3. Individual practice requires memorization of the entire sequence of movements. Once memory obstacles subside, your mind is then much more able to encompass the nuances of the movements. Surmounting this hurdle leads to greater progress.

How Long Should You Practice?

As a beginner, my enthusiasm was so intense that I frequently practiced past the point of diminishing returns. Presently, my enthusiasm is at least as intense, but it has mellowed with an awareness that excesses are contrary to the ideas of balance and proportion embodied in T'ai Chi Ch'uan. Once diminishing returns occur, I go on to other things. I know that there is a natural rate of progress that cannot be forced.

Indoor or Outdoor Practice?

An important advantage of outdoor practice is the presence of fresh air, natural light, and the sounds, sights, and smells of nature. However, not everyone is able to find such a practice site. Many practitioners live in a region where, outdoors, they are exposed to polluted air, harsh and incessant sounds of barking dogs, booming box radios, traffic, and jet planes, overbearing onlookers, uneven ground, extremes of temperatures, and annoying insects. Everything should be taken into account when deciding where to practice.

One of my students practiced outdoors every day, regardless of the weather. He said that at first it was very difficult during cold weather, but he was gradually able to feel comfortable. The ability of the body to adapt to external extremes is a valuable asset.

Time of Day for Practice

Traditionally, T'ai Chi Ch'uan is practiced at sunrise and at sunset. At these times, the ch'i emanated by the earth, trees, and heaven is considered to be the strongest. However, it is good to practice at any time except just after a meal (see "Eating Before or After Practice," later in this chapter) or, for male practitioners, immediately after sexual intercourse involving an ejaculation. The time of day to practice is totally up to the student, who should experiment with finding a personal "best time." A commitment to practice at that time every day reduces lost days and intensifies the focus during practice.

One good time to practice is during a creative endeavor, when a prolonged impasse is encountered. Often, at that time, we feel that we must struggle on. However, one round of T'ai Chi Ch'uan restores energy and objectivity. When the endeavor is resumed, the time invested is usually saved many times over.

Self-Discipline

There is a thin line between forcing and coddling oneself. On one hand, we would like things to happen naturally and spontaneously. However, most of us find that even that to which we are committed can go by the wayside without some resolve. I can remember standing on the edge of the swimming pool in my bathing suit for quite some time because I dreaded the initial chill of the water. There are times when we must give ourselves an initial push. Usually, that is all that is needed.

Fear of Mistakes

In many cases, mistakes can have serious consequences. We know this danger and fear mistakes. When we do make a mistake, we feel guilty and remorseful, and some of us even punish ourselves in one way or another.

However, mistakes during the learning process are natural and do not have bad consequences. In fact, they are valuable (if not essential) opportunities for learning. Because the fear of making mistakes has been so ingrained in us by schooling, etc., many of us avoid making mistakes to an extent that severely stunts the learning process.

In the practice of T'ai Chi Ch'uan there are very few mistakes that are so serious that repeating them for one week will become any sort of problem. Cheng Man-ch'ing said, "Repeating a fundamental error for more than *three years* makes it very hard to reverse." However, most students will fail to practice for fear of making an inconsequential mistake for only *one week*. I frequently hear beginning students say, "I didn't want to do it wrong, so I didn't practice." My answer is, "Do the best you can. There will be more that is correct than incorrect. You will be getting the benefits of what you are doing correctly. You will be relaxing, strengthening your legs, releasing your mind from mechanical thinking, and connecting your mind and body. Moreover, when you familiarize yourself with a move, during the next class, you will be much more likely to see what you are doing wrong and correct it. If you don't practice, you will keep making the same mistakes in class, and progress will be stunted."

The real mistake is not practicing for fear of making a mistake.

The Mind During Practice

Students will unhappily say, "My mind wanders during practice," or, "I can't seem to do a whole form without losing concentration." T'ai Chi Ch'uan has been called a "moving meditation," which implies that the mental state achieved is the same as or very similar to that during a sitting meditation. Many take this idea seriously enough to imbue their practice with a carry-over of the same mental focus that they associate with sitting meditation. Some who do sitting meditation believe that the mental repetition of a phrase or an idea will produce the desired effect. Others steadfastly fix their mind on one idea. While these techniques are important for building concentration and while concentration is a vital aspect of T'ai Chi Ch'uan, these techniques, if carried far enough, result in stagnant fixation—the very opposite of the basic principles of both sitting meditation and T'ai Chi Ch'uan.

In certain types of sitting meditation, the goal is for the mind to transcend the body. Here, the body is safe and quiet, and the main bodily activities that now occur are breathing, circulation of blood, functioning of the organs, etc., which are autonomic processes that do not require the mind. However, in practicing T'ai Chi Ch'uan, the mind is actively engaged in overseeing voluntary physical activities that involve judgment, coordination, balance, stepping, timing, and sensing gravity, air, the movements of others, spatial relationships of one's self to physical objects in the room, and the flow of ch'i. Therefore, it is inappropriate for the mind to leave the body under these conditions. The type of concentration required for purely mental activities during sitting meditation is different from the concentration required for the combined physical and mental activities of T'ai Chi Ch'uan.

The T'ai Chi Ch'uan movements themselves, plus their associated foci of awareness, provide a built-in mechanism that insures that benefits will be achieved without Herculean attempts to fix the mind on a particular idea or concept. Of course, it is valuable to achieve a continuing awareness of a particular theme or concept during a round of practice. For example, you can concentrate to advantage on sinking, rooting, breathing, stepping, relaxation, separation of yin and yang, or continuity. However, you need not always avoid a round on "automatic pilot," wherein your mind goes wherever it wants or merely savors the many principles brought to life through the movements.

Ways of Practicing

The practice of T'ai Chi Ch'uan can be likened to cleaning a house. For example, one should not go for more than a day without washing the dishes or putting dirty clothes in the hamper, etc. By the same token one should avoid letting more than one day go by without practice. However, one should not constantly worry about straightening things up. Every now and then focused attention must be paid, for instance, to cleaning out the attic or basement of a house. This focus corresponds to doing the form with special attention to one principle or theme. In this manner the depth of experience of doing the form increases with time. The result is a fulfillment that stems both from doing the form and a sense of being instrumental in a process of growth.

The following are a number of suggested themes for practice. Lest this list seem overwhelming, it should be noted that not more than one of these themes need be incorporated in any one practice session or series of sessions.

At different speeds. The question, "How fast should the form be practiced?" has no simple answer. On the one hand, for each practitioner, there is an optimal speed for cultivating the flow of ch'i and harmonizing the breath with the movements. On the other hand, there are different benefits corresponding to different speeds.

While a very slow speed may not conduce to the flow of ch'i or to an ideal coordination of breathing with the movements, it provides the opportunity for the mind to encompass more. A slow speed is good for checking alignment, relaxation, synchronization, balance, separation of yin and yang, and the fidelity of postures and transitions. For this reason, beginners are especially encouraged to do the movements as slowly as possible. In doing the movements slowly, inaccuracies become more evident and are best remedied.

One way of doing the form is what I call *quasi static. Quasi* means almost, and *static* means *still.* Therefore, to do the form quasi statically means doing the form so slowly that there is almost no perceptible movement.

After the continuity and shape of the movements have become encompassed by the mind, the next step is to become aware of the circulation of the ch'i and the coordination of the breath with the movements. (See the discussion of "Breathing" in chapter 4.) After ch'i is experienced, the movements should be practiced at such a speed and in such a manner that optimize the circulation of ch'i.

At first, it is a major accomplishment to do the moves in such a way as to circulate the ch'i. Later, when circulation of ch'i becomes second nature, it is a good idea to gradually increase the speed without losing the integrity and continuity of the movements and the flow of ch'i. Eventually the movements can be done quickly, with the ch'i being the propelling agent.

Moving very quickly increases the risk that the principles will be violated. For that reason, a high speed brings out inaccuracies and fuzziness. The maximum speed that should be practiced is one that reveals errors but does not lead to a degradation of quality. All of the principles must be adhered to at a high speed. Increasing the speed in this manner will lead to a quicker focusing of the ch'i. The instantaneous focus of ch'i is required in an actual self-defense situation.

At home, you should experiment with all speeds. Of course, during a given round, the speed should not change except for the ebb and flow of each move. In class, the speed must be that of the group ("sticking"). By practicing at different speeds at home, you will be comfortable with whatever speed the leader selects even if that speed is not the optimal one for the circulation of your ch'i.

In summary, each speed of doing the form corresponds to a different idea and to a unique benefit. Therefore, it is good to vary the speed from round to round. However, during a given round, a consistent speed should be maintained.

Mirror image. At a certain point, a thoughtful student will wonder if it is a good idea to do the mirror image of the movements. When I had been with Professor Cheng several months, I innocently asked this question of one of the senior students. He immediately brought me to Professor Cheng, who was told through an interpreter, "This student wants to do the mirror image of the form." Professor Cheng was very concerned, and he carefully explained to me (through the interpreter) that the Yang family never allowed any of their students to do the mirror image of the form. The reason given for this was, "We are not the same on both sides, and the form is geared to take these differences into account. The liver is on the right side, the heart is more on the left, and the left lung is smaller than the right lung. Even left-handed people are stronger on the right side. All of the movements of the form take into account the differences between the two sides of the body and the way the ch'i flows. Doing the mirror image can make you sick!"

Professor Cheng, a world-famous practitioner of Chinese herbology and acupuncture (in addition to painting, T'ai Chi Ch'uan, and calligraphy), frequently alluded to the fact that the left lung was smaller and also told us not to sleep on our left side because it would be bad for that lung. Moreover, Cheng told us that the "Single Whip" posture was good for opening the right lung and that his teacher, Yang Cheng-fu, recommended this posture to him for his tuberculosis. While I cannot say that I have ever noticed any particular effect on my right lung from the single whip, there is no question in my mind that, when I lie on my left side, I feel a constriction of the left lung. However, I feel no similar constriction when I lie on my right side.

My present teacher, Harvey Sober, emphasizes learning everything equally on both sides as soon as possible. He feels that "the benefits of doing the mirror image far outweigh any minor and unlikely side effects." Many other teachers would concur with Sober.

Cheng man-ch'ing's short form, presented in the Appendix of this book is intended by him to be done only on one side under the direction of a competent teacher. Practitioners should not attempt to do the other side until they are sufficiently familiar with the natural flow of ch'i that they can tell if it is disrupted.

Blindfolded or in the dark. Our sense of balance is determined by three mechanisms. (1) We attain physical balance mainly through the motion and pressure of fluid in the semicircular canals, which are part of the organs of hearing. (2) Visually noting the apparent movement of different objects in the background provides an extremely sensitive indicator of movement away from equilibrium. (3) The feeling of the ground against our feet tells us when we are losing our balance.

By eliminating the visual aspect, we must rely on the other two mechanisms, which then become more effectively trained (see "Balance" in chapter 3).

Compressed. When doing T'ai Chi Ch'uan alone, it is useful to know how to modify the moves so that they fit into a limited available space. Or, when doing the form in a group in close proximity to others, it frequently occurs that those whose stepping or whose concept of the moves is different from your own may start to close in on your space. Here, it is desirable to be able to modify the movements of the form to prevent interference with others. Any modification must be done without losing continuity of movement.

Form compression is accomplished through the following modification of the process of stepping as taught to me by William C. C. Chen:

When a space problem is anticipated, merely place the stepping foot wherever you like. Then shift 100% of the weight to that foot, and reposition the other foot in its proper relationship to the first foot. Next distribute the weight as it should be for that posture. (The final stance must not be affected.)

For example, imagine that, in doing "Brush Knee Left," there is an obstacle forward and to the left. Thus, there is insufficient space for the left foot to step as usual into a 70-30 posture. Instead of the left foot stepping forward and a shoulder width to the left, that foot can be judiciously placed short of its usual placement (or anywhere else, for that matter). Next, as the posture is being completed, the right foot must be relocated to compensate for the short step. Relocation is done by momentarily shifting 100% of the weight onto the left foot and lifting and repositioning the right foot to give the final "Brush Knee" posture the correct length and width.

Or, for example, in "Repulse Monkey," if there is no room to take steps backward, step the forward foot only as far back as the rear foot, and then move the rear foot forward to its usual position in that posture.

With some practice, it is possible to do the complete form in a space four feet by four feet, automatically adjusting as the need arises.

Compressing the form not only helps to solve the practical problem of lack of space but also develops judgment, visualization, and a sense of spatial and temporal relations. For example, when doing T'ai Chi Ch'uan in a group, it becomes necessary to observe the need in others to compress their movements and thereby anticipate the need to correspondingly compress your own movements inconspicuously, without interrupting the flow.

A few years ago my students and I successfully did the complete short form, each of us on the top of a circular table four feet in diameter. And, because of our concern that stepping too close to the edge might tip over the table, we actually stayed well within the four-foot-by-four-foot boundary.

A good way to practice compressing the form is to lay out a square on the floor with string.

Expanded. There is an optimal length for each 70-30 stance, as described in chapter 7. However, in a self-defense situation it is not always possible to step in such a manner that the weight is not committed. Therefore, it is of value to practice taking a larger-than-normal step. Because such stepping makes the final stance unnaturally long, the rear foot is allowed to slide a corresponding amount. This type of stepping is illustrated by many of the movements of the Two-Person (San Shou) Form.

Extra low. Every now and then it is good to do a round of the form, sinking the weight totally. Most teachers of T'ai Chi Ch'uan place a major emphasis on sinking. The more the upper body relaxes, the greater the stress on the legs. Thus, the strength of the legs is a limiting factor in the degree of relaxation of the upper body. By strengthening the legs to withstand stress, the upper body becomes increasingly able to relax. Of course, strong legs are also very important for stability (rooting) and for the circulation of the blood.

The student will find that by doing the form very low, benefits will be achieved that are similar to those of doing calisthenics such as push-ups, sit-ups, chin-ups, etc. However, because, during T'ai Chi Ch'uan practice, the leg muscles are stressed at their full elongation, they will become strong without the loss of flexibility and without the abnormal development caused by calisthenics. Not only that, but, the stress on the bones will strengthen them and increase their density.

On different surfaces. The elastic and frictional properties of wood make a level, polished, wooden floor the ideal surface on which to practice. Concrete floors do not flex and are hard on the feet. With certain footwear, such as rope-soled "kung fu" slippers, rugs provide a disagreeably large amount of friction, making pivoting hard. Rugs with foam underneath make balance more difficult. Uneven surfaces such as grass, sand, or earth challenge you to adapt to constantly changing conditions. It is good to get used to practicing on all manner of surfaces.

In different directions or places. Beginners often find a change of starting direction to be quite disorienting. Once students get home after a class, they tend to forget the movements they just learned. This disorientation is partly because the visual cues are now different. The movements learned were associated with visual memories of surroundings rather than their having been independently conceptualized. For this reason it is very important to practice as soon as possible after a class. The student should occasionally attempt to do the form in an unfamiliar direction or in varied surroundings.

It is important for the teacher to give the student an opportunity during class for individual practice. To some extent, this simulates conditions outside class, where there will not be others from whom to copy. If the teacher does not formally give the students an opportunity to practice on their own, the teacher will usually not object to the student occasionally practicing individually, off to one side.

Alternatively, one can practice mentally, as described next.

In your mind. Going through the movements mentally while you are standing, sitting, or lying down is especially useful. If nothing else, it challenges and thereby improves concentration. It is much harder to sustain concentration while lying down or sitting than when actually doing the movements.

For beginning students, visualization is a highly recommended tool for practice—not only for remembering the sequence of moves but also for eliminating errors and discovering states of tension. The state of general relaxation normally achieved when sitting or lying down leads to an awareness of tensions that can go unnoticed during ordinary practice.

Visualization is an important way of practicing when you are sick and lack the strength to do the form all the way through. A number of years ago I was so sick (104° F fever for one week) that I was barely able to get out of bed. Of course, I attempted to practice the form every day. I was only able to do the first section before I was completely exhausted and had to lie down on the floor to rest. However, this practice plus visualizing myself doing the entire form was very valuable—if only because I felt that I was able to do something constructive for myself in my highly weakened condition.

I do not know whether it was this practice, the fact that I fasted, or the stepped-up elimination of toxins as a result of my fever, but, when my fever went down I felt better than I had for a number of years. Naturally, it took a few months for my full energy to return.

Robert Smith[2] tells about a bedridden, nearly paralyzed person who was not expected to survive. "A (T'ai Chi Ch'uan) teacher came and did the exercise as the invalid looked on." The patient recovered, and "In three months he returned to work." This story illustrates the powerful non-physical healing aspect of T'ai Chi Ch'uan.

Stopping and repeating a move or part of a move. While it is of great value to do an entire form without interruption, sometimes it is better to stop at a point where a violation of the principles is discovered. Then, that defect can be isolated, worked on, and eliminated.

Each of the individual movements of the form or small sections of the form can be isolated and repeatedly practiced as an exercise. Such repetition highlights features of a movement and allows the frequent examination and refinement of those features. At the same time, the practitioner still receives most of the usual benefits of doing the entire form.

During practice, musicians frequently isolate and repeatedly play a small passage of a musical composition. They do not need to start each time at the beginning but choose any appropriate place. T'ai Chi Ch'uan practitioners should follow this approach. When practicing a given movement, it is best to start by assuming the final position of the previous posture, first checking the integrity of that posture.

An individual move such as "Beginning" can easily be repeated any number of times in succession since it starts and ends in exactly the same position. Moves such as "Rollback and Press," "Withdraw and Push," "Punch," "Descending Single Whip," and "Bend the Bow to Shoot the Tiger" do not start and end in exactly the same position. However, each of these moves can be individually repeated by simply adding a small variation that bridges the discrepancy between the beginning and end.

"Pivot on Heel and Kick with Heel" can be repeated in each of the eight directions: N, NE, E, SE, S, SW, W, and NW (although not in that order). If the kick is normally done in the easterly direction, one round involves kicking sequentially in each of the eight directions E, NW, S, NE, W, SE, N, and SW. This sequence stems from the fact that each pivot rotates the body leftward by 135°. After a round is completed, you automatically face the starting direction again. This exercise builds balance, spatial relations, and strength of legs. It will be discovered that smoothly completing one round without hesitating or losing your balance is quite demanding.

Two sequential moves such as "Hands Playing the P'i P'a" and "Brush Knee" can be repeated as a pair. Other sequential pairs that are useful to repeat include "Raise Hands" and "Shoulder Strike," "Fair Lady Left" and "Fair Lady Right," "Step Back to Ride The Tiger" and "Turn to Sweep the Lotus," and "Separate Right Foot" and "Separate Left Foot."

A larger sequence of moves or even an entire section of the form may be repeated. Rather than pausing between repetitions, it is better to employ smooth transitions.

A number of moves in the form occur in succession on both the right and left side. Examples of this are "Ward off," "Repulse Monkey," "Four Corners," and "Brush Knee." Such moves may be repeated many more times than the standard number. Also, if you decide to do the mirror image of other moves that are normally done on one side only, a possible way of practicing is to take such a move and create an alternating right-left sequence. For this sequence to work, the movement should be one that starts with the weight on one foot and ends with the weight on the opposite foot. A good example of such a move is "Single Whip," which starts with 70% of the weight on the right foot and ends with 70% of the weight on the left foot. Other movements that lend themselves to repeated mirrored alternation are "Shoulder Strike," "Diagonal Flying," "Hands Playing the P'i P'a," and "Turn to Sweep the Lotus."

It should be noted that while "Cloud Hands" has a right and left version, these are not true mirror images of each other since, in each version, the stepping is in the same direction.

The names of the postures should be committed to memory to facilitate later reference to a given position. A list of the names of the postures of Cheng Man-ch'ing's short form can be found at the beginning of the Appendix.

Emphasizing a principle or idea. An entire form or section of a form may be done while concentrating on one of the following concepts:

- Stepping like a cat
- Breathing
- Circulation of ch'i
- Relaxation of shoulders, elbows, abdomen, face, neck, trunk, feet, and legs
- Continuity of movement
- Yin and Yang (empty and full)
- Alignment of arches, ankles, knees, pelvis, head, wrist, etc. (knees not buckling in, "beauteous" wrist)
- Coordination of circular movements with the shifting of the weight
- Circles
- Filling each move
- Centering of the joints, and optimizing the space between fingers and between arms and body (see also chapter 5)
- Not turning the head
- Keeping an even level (sinking during transitions)
- Not twisting the body
- Letting the eyes liquefy—taking in the full 180-degree panorama without "looking"
- Cultivating a feeling of well being, inner peace, love of nature, and gratitude for being healthy and having the life force permeate your being

Supplementary Exercises

Movements other than those in the form can be practiced to remedy a weakness, study alignment, or heal an injury. Here is an exercise, taught by Professor

Cheng, that is excellent for strengthening the legs, developing balance and root, and bringing a lot of blood and healing energy to the knees: Stand on one leg with the weighted foot at an angle of 45° to 90° with the forward direction. Then move the heel of the empty foot forward in a vertical circle by lifting it, extending it outward, and then moving it downward, keeping it extended. After a round of thirty-six repetitions and a brief rest, switch sides. It will be found that doing a full round is quite demanding. Many practitioners will need to work up to thirty-six repetitions over a period of time. Elderly or weak people can do this exercise holding on to a piece of furniture until sufficient strength and balance are developed. The correct alignment of the leg and foot is achieved when the center line of the 100%-weighted foot is in the same plane as that formed by the ankle, knee, and thigh joint of that leg (see "Alignment," chapter 5).

One exercise that is commonly practiced is to stand on one leg for increasingly extended periods of time. This exercise can be done while standing in line or waiting for a bus or a train. While standing on one leg, the other leg is allowed to touch the floor but with no pressure (empty). You should practice sinking the weight into the rooted leg. Special attention must be paid to the looseness and alignment of both the upper body and the legs. With practice, you will be gradually able to increase the maximum time spent on each leg. After rooting on one side, the thigh muscles of the fatigued leg should be encouraged to relax by lightly kicking the heel downward in the air a few times.

Another similar exercise is to stand for increasingly long periods of time in the 70-30 stance (see chapter 7). Again, sinking the weight, and attention to correct alignment are of great importance here.

Exercises for Improving Balance

Just doing the T'ai Chi Ch'uan form according to the principles will automatically improve your balance; namely, stepping must be done without committing the weight (separation of yin and yang), and the weight of the body must be allowed to sink into the legs (being rooted). However, the following are some exercises that can greatly accelerate the rate of progress:

1. An important facet of balance is the correct alignment of the feet, ankles, knees, pelvis, spine, and head, as previously discussed in the chapter on "alignment" (chapter 5).

   The next exercise will be found useful in discovering and sensitizing you to the precise location of the centers of the feet. As a by-product, this exercise will also fine-tune the alignment of arches, ankles, and knees:

   While standing in a fifty-fifty stance, rock forward and backward on both feet. Feel the center of the pressure distribution alternately moving forward and backward from the center of each foot. After rocking for a while, gradually decrease the amount of movement, sustaining your awareness of the centers of the feet and the movements toward and away from these centers. Next, move the knees toward and away from each other, feeling the center of the pressure distribution alternately moving inward and outward from the centers of the feet. Again, gradually decrease the amount of movement, sustaining your awareness of the centers of the feet and the movements toward and away from these centers. When the pressure is centered on the feet in both forward and sideways directions, not only will stability be optimal, but the alignment of the arches, ankles, and knees will also be correct.

2. One of the most important aspects of balance is the principle of "sung." When the upper body becomes relaxed, and the weight is allowed to sink into the legs, it is as though the center of mass of the body were below the floor (see the section on "Balance" in chapter 3 for a discussion of center of mass). Of course, while it is physically impossible for the center of mass of an inanimate object to be below its lowest material point, for a living structure, it is possible to create a dynamic condition in which the center of mass appears to be below the ground. That is, when an opponent tries to uproot you with a push, by achieving a state of sung and correctly neutralizing, you can give the pushing person the distinct feeling that your center of mass is below the ground. It is said that the goal is to achieve a center of mass six feet below the ground!

   Caution: It is essential that correct alignment of arches, ankles, and knees be achieved before gradually allowing sung to permeate the lower body. Otherwise, injury can occur. Any lingering pain in the knees is a danger sign.

3. Select a small section of the form such as the two successive moves, "White Crane Spreads Wings" and "Brush Knee." Do these as 100%-weighted moves as follows: Assume the "White Crane" posture, with the right foot at 90° to the forward direction. Instead of touching the ball of the empty left foot to the ground, lift the left knee, as in "Golden Cock Stands on Right Leg." Instead of stepping into "Brush Knee," continue to suspend the left knee, and repeat the sequence. At first, only one repetition will be very tiring. Later, the number of repetitions can be increased. After a sufficient number of repetitions of the sequence, place the left foot at 90° to the forward direction and do the same sequence of repetitions on the other side.

4. First do the entire form in the dark or with eyes closed. As balance improves, isolate a series of moves such as the ones just described, and then do them on one leg. Because the visual aspect of balance tends to dominate, doing movements without using the eyes (in the dark or with eyes closed) increases the challenge to the remaining senses.

Use of a Mirror

Watching yourself in a mirror while doing the T'ai Chi Ch'uan form has value but should not be done consistently. It is occasionally important to notice certain objective details such as leaning, committing of the weight, incorrect alignment, and integrity of the postures. However, the correct execution of all these details should eventually stem from an inner rather than external awareness.

If a mirror is not available, a single, lamp will produce a well-defined shadow on the wall.

Use of Music or a Metronome

Some practitioners of T'ai Chi Ch'uan use music in different ways. One concept is that, in a self-defense situation, you must move to the timing of the opponent. Therefore it is considered to be of value to practice the form to a beat. This beat can be provided by music or the regular click of a metronome.

One of my students, whose prior teacher used a metronome, had difficulty in doing the form to her own inner flow. It took her about a year of practicing without the metronome to get its sound out of her mind's ear. Because there are enough foci of timing provided by the already existing internal and external dynamics of the form, imposing an arbitrary beat is unnecessary if not substantially limiting.

Doing the form with music in the background (rather than to its beat) is certainly enjoyable and can add a dimension to one's practice. However, such practice should be balanced by at least an equal period of practice without any music.

As a physics teacher, I have encountered many students who claimed that they could concentrate on their homework while listening to music. I find that when I try to do two things simultaneously, each detracts from the other. When I listen to music, I want to give it my full attention, and when I do physics, the less extraneous sensory input to my brain, the better it functions. With regard to T'ai Chi Ch'uan, each practitioner will have to decide this issue individually.

Practice in Everyday Life

Professor Cheng used to say that mere practice of the form is superfluous when everything a practitioner does is in accordance with the principles of T'ai Chi Ch'uan. As a result of these words, early on in my study of T'ai Chi Ch'uan, I became inspired to infuse every action in my daily life with the T'ai Chi Ch'uan principles.

For example, when I drove my car, I practiced holding the steering wheel so lightly that I could feel the effect of every change in the road surface. After a while, I was able to feel the slightest tendency of my car to skid on wet or icy roads and could react immediately. I also practiced moving my hand from the steering wheel to the horn and back. This practice developed a very fast "horn reflex."

I used opportunities, such as standing on a check-out line in a store, to root by standing on one leg while relaxing the upper body. I also practiced walking in such a manner that I did not commit my weight to a foot before feeling the ground underneath. This practice once saved me from what would have been a serious accident. I was in the loft of a lumber yard looking for an exotic wood.

Suddenly I became aware that my stepping foot was not touching the floor. I looked at the place where I was stepping. I saw that, had I committed my weight to that foot prematurely, I would have fallen through an opening that was a dozen feet above the concrete floor below. Shaken but safe, I said to myself, "That's T'ai Chi Ch'uan."

After a few years of doing T'ai Chi Ch'uan, I began to notice that I was doing many things differently than before. On arising from a night's sleep, I found myself gliding out of bed, my feet meeting the floor as in doing the form. I noticed that when sitting down in a chair, I automatically used the principle analogous to that of not committing my weight when stepping. While I still am far from the point where *everything* I do is in accordance with the T'ai Chi Ch'uan principles, I see that more and more, the principles have permeated my daily life.

The T'ai Chi Ch'uan principles need not always be applied to physical events but can be used in human interactions. The following story will illustrate this application: I was shopping in a supermarket, and, because I had only three items, I went to the line with a sign, "10 items or less." (Grammatically, the sign should have read, "10 items or *fewer.*") Ahead of me was a woman who had many more than ten items. I could see that, should anyone challenge her, she was preparing to group the groceries into two purchases, each of which would contain fewer than ten items. Avoiding a confrontation, I simply said to her, "I have only three items. Would you mind if I went ahead?" Relieved, she graciously invited me to go ahead, and I thanked her.

The highest use of T'ai Chi Ch'uan is to neutralize a potential confrontation in such a manner that all concerned are benefited and uplifted.

Eating Before or After Practice

Neither meditation nor exercise should ever be done on a full stomach. Since T'ai Chi Ch'uan is both meditation and exercise, this caution holds doubly. During digestion, the blood becomes channeled to the digestive organs. Digestion involves (a) glandular secretions produced from blood and (b) muscular contractions that require stepped-up circulation of blood to the stomach. Thus the amount of blood available to the brain and skeletal muscles is reduced. The reduction of blood to the brain affects mental concentration. The competition between the muscles and the stomach results in neither of these doing an optimal job.

I have found that merely eating a piece of fruit before practice produces a just-noticeable adverse affect on my balance and concentration. Aside from hindering practice, eating a full meal before can result both in gastric discomfort and a strain on the heart.

While many practitioners eat immediately after practicing, doing so is not a good idea for the following reason: During practice there is a stepped-up elimination of toxins from the leg muscles, organs, and deeper tissues of the body. The kidneys are especially active in this cleansing process, as can be verified by observing that after practice, your urine will frequently be dark and concentrated—a sign that poisons have been eliminated.

If no meal is taken after practice, the cleansing continues. However, once the body is required to engage in the digestion of food, again, the blood goes to the stomach rather than moving toxins from the leg muscles to the organs of elimination.

Experiment by paying close attention to the effects over a twenty-four hour period of either eating or not eating immediately after intense practice. Then note the quality of your sleep, the presence or absence of subsequent soreness, and the degree that you sense a feeling of well-being.

If you feel that it is absolutely necessary to eat before or after practice, then eat a piece of fresh fruit. For some reason, eating a banana after strenuous practice seems to ward off soreness the next day. Since there is potassium loss in muscles during exercise, it is commonly thought that the potassium in the bananas replaces the potassium lost by the muscles. While bananas are not low in potassium, they are not unusually high in that nutrient (370 mg/100 g, which is the same as that in cooked beef).[3] Therefore, the reason for the benefit may be more complex than potassium replacement alone.

Aspirin, taken just before a workout seems to have a beneficial effect, possibly because it thins the blood and thus helps circulation. Aspirin for a fever is an entirely different matter; anything that suppresses the body's natural function is to be totally avoided.

"Cool-Down" of the Leg Muscles

After strenuous T'ai Chi Ch'uan practice, the muscles of the legs need to continue to move so that the elimination of toxins can occur. The worst thing to do after a practice session is to drive an automobile for an extended period of time, with the legs bent and motionless. If you must drive after heavy practice, it is a good idea to stop the car a few times during the trip and get out and move around.

In my very first class with Professor Cheng, he taught us the kidney rub, which is very important for the cleansing of the leg-muscle tissues (see chapter 9).

TEACHERS
Choosing a Teacher

While the choice of a teacher is highly individual, there are some general guidelines.

Bear in mind that some teachers have a policy of not advertising and keep a "low profile." Such a teacher may not have a formal school but teach students in relatively small groups in adult-education centers, places of worship, or in their own homes. Usually, such teachers do not solely rely on teaching T'ai Chi Ch'uan for a living. The way to locate low-profile teachers is through word of mouth, demonstrations they present, or articles or books that they write.

Once teachers and schools are found, the next step is to call each teacher and ask whether it is possible to visit a class. It is standard policy for a teacher to extend an invitation to observe or take part in a class at no charge. You may visit as many different schools as you want but not more than once each.

Some teachers are very formal; others are informal. Some schools are competitive; others are not. Some teachers require students to wear a uniform or a logo-imprinted tee shirt, whereas other teachers encourage their students to wear what they want. These are all policies that are subject to personal preference.

When you are visiting a school, you should notice the student-student and student-teacher rapport or absence thereof. Notice if the students seem to be learning or if they have previously learned anything. Are the students enjoying what they are doing? Are more-advanced movements taught, such as the double-edged sword, broadsword, or two-person forms? Does the teacher display knowledge of anything other than T'ai Chi Ch'uan?

Some teachers insist that new students start in a class solely for beginners. Other teachers allow beginners to be in the same class with more advanced students. Some teachers teach the long form, and others teach a shortened version. Each of these policies has advantages and disadvantages and should not be an important criterion for deciding upon a teacher. Teachers vary greatly in their approach, and the beginner must decide on a teacher in a highly subjective manner.

A factor of substantial importance is a teacher's lineage. Did the teacher study under one or more recognized masters?

Methods of T'ai Chi Ch'uan Teachers

Students of a martial art initially tend to carry over their expectations from previous schooling. Since martial arts teachers transfer knowledge in such different ways, often the student will emphasize the wrong things in practicing or miss essential details. Here are some of the ways that knowledge is transferred:

1. The teacher will go over a concept or action, have students work on it in class, and tell them to practice it at home. In the next class the teacher will go over it again, refining, correcting, and adding. One problem with this method is that some students will erroneously feel that the practice at home is not necessary, since so much time is devoted to repetition in class.

2. The teacher will show something but not necessarily give students a chance to practice it in class. There may not even be an allusion to it during the next class. One possible reason for this is that the teacher does not want to coddle students but wants them to take the initiative. Or, it may be that the teacher is tired that day and forgets to follow through. In any case, the student should follow through. After class, a student who is really excited about what is being taught will automatically review the class mentally and follow up on these things through devoted practice. Jotting down concise reminders during or immediately after class is extremely helpful. It is wise to keep a notebook exclusively for these notes.

3. The teacher will show something without even being conscious of it. For example, my present teacher, Harvey Sober, would occasionally do Pa-Kua Chang[4] moves off on the side while the class was doing other movements. I observed this out of the corner of my eye so frequently that I found myself spontaneously doing these moves at times. There are other less obvious instances where the teacher will make a subliminal impression on the student through repeated movements or gestures.

4. It is possible to learn from a teacher whose identity is completely unknown to the student. This may sound unbelievable, so prepare yourself for something strange. The teacher may be a consciousness that may or may not even reside in a living body. The teacher may have died and not yet have been reborn. Or, the teacher may at present be a child who, in a past life, attained some sort of mastery. It may be that the teacher had a strong connection with the student but passed on. Or, the teacher may have had no connection in this life but, rather, in past lives. Or, the connection may even be much less fathomable. The student may not even be consciously aware of being taught through "spirit." Such an awareness, however, can make the process more efficient. If the instruction is coming, for example, through dreams (as mine most often does), the student can do various things to increase the likelihood that contact will be made and that what is received is consciously retained upon awakening. Future contacts can be initiated by consciously desiring the contact to be made. Retention can be increased by an awareness that an important process is taking place. The knowledge that you are being helped in spirit adds an extra keenness to your receptivity.

5. Occasionally a student will ask a question, and the teacher will seem to answer a different question. One possibility, of course, is that the teacher did not understand the question. However there are other possibilities. The student may not realize that his question was, in fact, answered. Or, perhaps the teacher understood the question but preferred to answer a different question—one that the teacher felt should have been asked. In any case, the student should temporarily forego the need to have the teacher address what was originally asked and be receptive to what the teacher says. The original question can always be rethought and asked again at a later date.

6. Teachers will frequently correct a student's mistakes much more often than they commend the student. The teacher assumes that the student is working for self-cultivation rather than for praise. Students who expect their accomplishments to be acknowledged should not get discouraged by the teacher's lack of verbal reassurance. Rather, they should channel their disappointment into a resolve to build an inner strength that does not require the approval of others.

When I started T'ai Chi Ch'uan, I was extremely sensitive to criticism. Seeing my resistance, Cheng's senior students, who assisted in teaching, soon refrained from giving me corrections. After a short period of time,

I realized that corrections were essential to my progress. I then started to elicit corrections, and these were soon plentiful. Even though I still did not like to hear that I was making an error, the predominating feeling was now one of genuine gratitude.

Some teachers feel that it is their duty to throw obstacles in the path of the student. Since natural obstacles abound even under optimal conditions, teacher-contrived obstacles are unnecessary.

7. Each teacher has a different background and, consequently, a different emphasis. Cheng Man-ch'ing's major emphasis on the health aspects of T'ai Chi Ch'uan was because it saved his life. He was not expected to live past his twenties because of tuberculosis. Harvey Sober emphatically states that he owes being alive to the study of martial arts. When the doctors told him that he was "terminal" with ulcerative colitis, Sober's teacher, Chen Mai-Shou, told him, "If you stay here (in the hospital), you will die. I want you to go home immediately and do what I say." The breathing exercises that Sober did saved his life. It is no wonder that breathing is strongly emphasized in his teaching. Elaine Summers, with whom I studied "Kinetic Awareness," had advanced arthritis. Her emphasis on the alignment of joints stemmed from her own painful experience, which allowed her to sensitively distinguish minute differences in alignment. While I never studied with T. T. Liang or Benjamin Lo, I know that each of them began T'ai Chi Ch'uan because of failing health, and they managed to become super-normal in the aspect of original limitation. Benjamin Lo started T'ai Chi Ch'uan as a young man because of a crippling disability of his legs. Presently in his sixties, his legs are stronger than those of most high-level practitioners. It is quite important for the student to be aware that the teacher has a particular background and corresponding emphasis and to put what is taught in the proper perspective.

When a teacher teaches a number of different things, the student is best off pursuing that in which the teacher is most interested at that time. When I attended City College around 1960, I was one of a number of students who "majored" in a particular teacher, Professor Irani. Irani's lectures were so stimulating that whenever possible, we would take or sit in on every course that he taught, regardless of the course title. For example, Professor Irani's elementary logic classes would be sprinkled with philosophy majors who had taken and mastered elementary logic years before but wanted to hear his inimitable and fascinating digressions, analogies, and insights. His digressions would lead to digressions within digressions, etc. However, Irani would always amaze us with the brilliance of his mind by never losing track of where he was and by beautifully tying up all of the ideas he presented.

The most important things that are learned from a teacher are to experience, emphasize, discover, and revere what the teacher has experienced, emphasized, discovered, and revered. The subject matter taught should be regarded mainly as a vehicle rather than as an end in itself. When diminishing returns are reached in the learning process, then you are better off seeking a different teacher.

The best teachers continually grow and expand at a sufficient rate that diminishing returns for students are delayed.

Asking Questions in Class

As a teacher of physics and of T'ai Chi Ch'uan, I have come to realize the effect on the learning process of students asking the proper questions. Moreover, as a student for an even longer period of time, I have experienced the asking of many questions by both fellow students and myself.

A teacher can be compared to a bell. For a bell to sound, it must be properly activated.

It has been my experience that most good teachers are motivated more by the interest and development of their students than anything else. Conversely, nothing can undermine a teacher more than students who are either uninterested or incapable of developing.

Students, on the other hand, tend to underestimate their effect upon the teacher, whom they tend to regard as immutable. Each student should therefore strive to become responsible for bringing out the highest level of the teacher.

Asking questions must not be contrived and, therefore, there are no fixed rules. However, keeping the following points in mind may be of some help.

1. Formulate each question to be clear and direct. Avoid spontaneous questions that have not been sufficiently thought out.

2. Do not use the opportunity to ask a question primarily to call attention to yourself or to exhibit your insight or understanding. It is permissible to ask a question to which you feel you know the answer if the motive is to verify or expand your knowledge. However, it is not appropriate to ask such a question for the purpose of showing off your knowledge.

3. Ask at the right time. Try to wait for an opportunity that does not involve an interruption of the teacher's train of thought or the flow of the class.

4. Do not feel stupid if a question falls flat on its face. Rather, analyze, without blame, how that question should have been asked.

5. If you ask the teacher a question after class, be prepared to terminate the communication as soon as the question is answered, unless the teacher demonstrates a keen desire to continue the communication. It is unfair to drain the teacher's energy.

Attitude Toward The Teacher

Even though T'ai Chi Ch'uan is very relaxed and informal, some basic rules apply.

1. When the teacher chooses a student with whom to demonstrate a certain push-hands or self-defense concept, it is not appropriate to try to test the teacher under these conditions, unless specifically requested to do so. This is because the teacher is concentrating on teaching rather than on

defending against an unexpected attack. In fact, an unexpected attack might evoke a sudden reflex action on the part of the teacher, resulting in injury to student or teacher. More likely, because the teacher has the student's safety uppermost in mind, the teacher will protect the student by not reacting, thereby causing the mistaken impression that the teacher was ineffectual. The best interests of all are served when the demonstrating student cooperates to illustrate what the teacher is showing.

I cannot help but recall one incident when Professor Cheng was demonstrating a push-hands concept to the class. At one point he stopped and said something in Chinese to the non-Chinese-speaking student with whom he was demonstrating. This utterance was translated as, "Please let go of my whiskers." (Professor Cheng had a long wispy beard that the student was inadvertently pulling.)

2. While teachers may become fond of their students, experienced T'ai Chi Ch'uan teachers will not become emotionally entangled with their students. Even if a student of long standing leaves, there is no attachment. By the same token, students must avoid becoming emotionally entangled with their teacher.

3. There is no teacher without faults, but students tend to see (or want to see) their teacher as perfect. The result is that students tend to copy everything about the teacher, including evident faults. The other extreme is for the student to become highly disillusioned with the teacher as soon as a fault emerges. The best approach is to be aware of the teacher's faults and copy the good things only.

"Perfect" Masters

There are differing interpretations of what constitutes a *master* of T'ai Chi Ch'uan. In any case, it is certain that there is no such thing as a *perfect master.* The very concept of a perfect master is limiting to students. When students think that the teacher is perfect, not only will they be blind to the teacher's inevitable faults, but, worse, they will copy these faults, thinking that the faults are correct actions.

One puzzling occurrence is the frequent contradiction between a teacher's actions in and out of class. In class, the teacher will display a continual uplifting series of insights into all manner of life situations. When a student has a problem or asks a question, the teacher will have a "master-level" response. However, in the teacher's own life, there will frequently be glaring actions that fall far short of the level displayed in class. Does this mean that the teacher is a hypocrite or a phony? Not necessarily. A better way of viewing this contradiction is to realize that in class the teacher acts as a medium through which knowledge of the ages passes to the *student and teacher alike.* Just because the spiritual level of that which passes through the teacher is not always manifested outside of class, this lack does not negate what passes through. Nor does it mean anything other than that teachers continue to aspire to that which they know or have access to but may not have mastered perfectly.

The main criterion is not whether the teacher is perfect but, rather, the extent to which the student is learning things of value and the manner in which these are assimilated.

ADVICE TO BEGINNERS

1. It is advisable for beginning students to be cautious about showing their movements or discussing the ideas of T'ai Chi Ch'uan with others. Naturally, you will want to share a new-found interest and hear others' opinions. However, this openness can be a mistake. Think of your connection with T'ai Chi Ch'uan as delicate and fragile. Exposing the flame of your new interest to the possible negativity of others who may not understand, may dampen that flame. When you ask others' opinions about an idea that you have, if your idea surpasses their thinking, their opinion will limit you. They will say, "That's impossible," or "That's ridiculous," or "You are wasting your time," and you will subconsciously believe them.

2. Try not to miss even one day of practice. If it is time to go to bed and you have not practiced that day, just remember that ten minutes of practice is worth more than an additional ten minutes of sleep. If you are too sick to do the form, visualize yourself doing it. If you do miss practice, do not allow this setback to discourage you. Simply return to practice.

3. Imitate your teacher's movements in every last detail. It is all too easy for a beginner to erroneously regard certain details as unimportant.

4. Put in your "back pocket" that which you already know. "An empty cup holds the most." Do not try to impress the teacher with your knowledge of other systems or teachings. When you begin with a new teacher or teaching, think of yourself as a beginner, no matter what your level is in other areas. A good teacher will quickly recognize and accommodate your capacity.

5. Do not miss a class unless it is absolutely necessary. Come to class even if you can only sit and watch.

THE LEARNING PROCESS

Goal Orientation

Our expectation of immediate results hampers the learning process to a great degree. When we constantly monitor our own "progress" and characterize its rate, we not only take away the joy of growth but can stunt it. Where did we learn to imbue learning with anxiety and negative thinking, and how can we reverse this trait? Consider the following:

Everyone has had the following experience in school: A teacher asks a question. A student's hand shoots up. The teacher calls on this student, who gives the answer before the other students have finished processing the question. Or, a teacher says, "The period is over; please hand in your test now." Many recurring experiences of this sort give students the impression that speed is one of the most important facets of learning. Why is speed so important?

Consider an assembly line on which automobiles are manufactured. Here partially completed automobiles move by, and each worker has a definite time period during which to install a particular part. The person who installs carburetors must get one in before the automobile moves out of range. The whole assembly line cannot be delayed just because a part is not completely installed, so the car moves on whether or not the installation is complete. If a worker is slow and is frequently responsible for incomplete installations, he will be replaced by a worker who *can* install a carburetor in the allotted time.

It is tacitly understood that school prepares us for the rigors of the machine-age, assembly-line workplace. We are taught to sit for many hours at a desk, just as we would in a clerical job. We learn how to control our impulses to move, talk, yawn, make sounds, stretch, drift off, etc. We learn that deadlines are sacred, and all of us are expected to reach the same stage of learning at the same time.

Much of this preparation does serve a legitimate purpose, since, to be intellectually productive, we need to be disciplined and able to meet deadlines.

The trouble begins when students tend to unfairly judge their own ability and progress in terms of an assembly line expectation. For example, the student who is a bit slower than the fastest student in the class will begin to feel inept, even if it is the case that he or she thinks more deeply, logically, and creatively—just slower. This student may be quite suited for a creative type of life's work. However, this student's growth is stunted when the learning process becomes permeated with the unarticulated and insidious dictates of industry—*insidious* because much of the educational process has come to be accepted and continued, without realization of its consequences, by students as well as teachers. Rather than savoring and cultivating the process by which knowledge is acquired, students tend to over-emphasize the end result such as a grade on a test or admission to a prestigious college. Unfortunately, the expectation of end results prompts students to constantly monitor their own "progress" and erroneously characterize its rate. Thus, students tend to lose the joy of growth and actually reduce their rate of learning.

How can students transcend this pitfall? We must start by becoming aware of and stripping away each and every negative message that we give ourselves while learning. For example, we have to stop saying—and even *thinking*—things such as, "I'm not really good at this," "I know I will never be able to do that as well as my classmate/sibling/parent/teacher can," or simply, "I'm stupid" or "I can't." We must learn to be infinitely patient with ourselves, unlike others may have been with us. When we are in a teaching or explaining position, we must develop patience with others. We must always emphasize process rather than results. The results will follow automatically. We need to cultivate pursuits that are so engrossing and stimulating that goals can be placed in the background rather than in our primary focus. Ideally, our pursuits should provide fascination and keen interest. They should also develop us and move us toward a goal that is intuitively felt but is not uppermost in our awareness. Eventually, each of us will develop patience, persistence, skill, health, self-awareness, awareness of others, etc., without much conscious thought focused on any of these as goals. The sheer enjoyment of learning should spur us on. The manifestation of our efforts should be a natural by-product of the learning process. Learning should be a joy.

A Tale about a Ruler and an Artist

Once, in ancient China, there was a ruler who wanted a painting of birds. He went to a famous artist and requested such a painting. The artist told the ruler that the painting would take one year.

Exactly one year later, the ruler went to the artist's house. He was invited in and was given refreshment. Then the artist took out some silk, started mixing his paint, and, within a short time, executed a magnificent painting of birds.

While impressed with the beauty of the painting, the ruler was perplexed. He said, "Why did you keep me waiting one year when such a painting is so easy to do?" In response, the artist took the ruler into the adjoining room. In that room were hundreds of paintings of birds.

The artist had devoted the whole year exclusively to the painting of birds. This preparation resulted in his being able to execute a flawless representation effortlessly in the presence of the ruler.

How is Progress Measured?

In certain activities, it is easy to measure progress. For example, in running, progress can be gauged in terms of distance and time. However, with T'ai Chi Ch'uan, it is hard for us to measure our progress. The benefits are subtle and not immediately noticed. Because of our preoccupation with goals, we tend to be very aware of external obstacles to progress and only see our inabilities, discouragements, and frustrations. Conversely, we tend not to notice our accomplishments and frequently take them totally for granted.

Imagine the frustration of a crawling child learning to walk. While frustrated, the child constantly sees others who are able to walk and intuitively understands that, with perseverance, success is assured. Eventually the infant is able to walk but then forgets what it was like not to walk. Each of us eventually walks without any conscious memory of that frustrating struggle.

Another aspect of the learning process is that the student measures progress in terms of the wrong parameters. Consider the following analogy of a student who needs to write a term paper on a certain subject. The student goes to the library to look up books on the subject and finds them unavailable at that branch. The student then goes home with the feeling that nothing has been accomplished. However, it was necessary for the student to have taken that first step before any true progress could be made. Therefore, that first step *was* progress, even though nothing tangible occurred.

In the case of the beginning T'ai Chi Ch'uan student, the inability to do a certain movement or to commit a certain sequence of moves to memory is regarded by that student as indicative of a lack of progress. However, it may be that many other things must first happen, but these things are neither visible, nor can they necessarily be articulated. It is all too easy to dwell on inabilities, which continuously emerge in the classroom atmosphere. However, every now and then, there may be a fleeting awareness of the progress made and the differences between past and present.

I encourage students who have studied T'ai Chi Ch'uan for about six months to visit a beginners' class. I do this for many reasons, one of which is that they get a glimpse of how far they have come since they, too, were rank beginners.

The best attitude to adopt is to view the learning process as analogous to "water wearing away rocks." In the study of geology we learn that mountains are changed to valleys by the process of erosion over millions of years. However, during one person's lifetime this effect is barely seen. The pursuit of any art of depth involves an analogous process. In the case of T'ai Chi Ch'uan, which alters one's mental preconceptions and the resulting bodily fixations and patterns of movement, progress may not be visible over a period short enough to be encompassed by the practitioner's mind.

The teacher is much more able to see the progress of the student because the teacher is not as emotionally involved and is more experienced at assessing the student's progress.

Perfectionism

One derogatory term that is applied to idealistic people is the word *perfectionist.* Perfectionists are thought to be doomed to a continually frustrating life of pursuing minutiae, thereby making everyone around them miserable. Perfectionists are considered to be neurotics, malcontents, and kill-joys—for themselves and others. While it is true that perfectionists frequently are unhappy people who make those around them miserable, this need not always happen, nor is perfectionism necessarily bad.

Those of us that come into this world with an ability to imagine the world in a better state—let alone a perfect state—come up against a tremendous resistance on the part of the majority of people who lack either the ability to conceive of anything better or the desire or patience to initiate it.

Those of us who are devoted to making things better than that which would satisfy the majority, are frequently burdened by our devotion. We are urged by others to give up our image of perfection (which we cannot), or we are punished when perfectionism is expressed. Eventually, perfectionists tend to become bitter and frustrated people who have given up all but the idea of perfection and the petty and compulsive expression of it.

However, think of the greatest works of art, technology, architecture, philosophy, etc. People such as Plato, Bach, Da Vinci, Michelangelo, etc., were perfectionists and contributed greatly to the upliftment of mankind. The difference between them and the stereotypical perfectionist is that these men were great geniuses who were able to accomplish what they set out to do. However, knowledge of their lives indicates that they had the same frustrations and difficulties as we do; it is just that they refused to let these stop them from actualizing their dreams. Each of us can bring out our own potential genius by focusing our creative energy with the persistence required.

My motto is, "Have an eye toward perfection, and have patience when perfection is not achieved."

Words and Speech

The spoken word has tremendous power. It is difficult to imagine what life would be like without speech. Words have the ability to communicate highly abstract thoughts with great efficiency. These days, there are numerous ways that speech can be almost instantaneously transmitted over large distances or stored and later played back.

Under some circumstances, though, speech has several negative aspects that are not commonly recognized. One such aspect is that words, by their very nature, limit our thinking.

Words embody concepts that are common to a large number of people. Otherwise, words would not have a communicative aspect. When ideas are expressed using words, those unique and highly individual thoughts, for which words are inadequate, become inhibited. That is, we implicitly know the limitations of verbal expression and thus, automatically tend to disregard certain delicate and unique thoughts because words cannot express them. This danger holds for people with a strong command of language as well as those with a limited command. The more we attempt to express thoughts using language, the better we get at minimizing those thoughts that are unique to us and inexpressible in words. This limitation not only applies to communication but, more importantly, to our thought processes.

Next, the words we use have embedded in them the distortions, misconceptions, biases, emotions, prejudices, etc., of others. When we use these words, we subtly accept to a certain degree the premises of the underlying distortions, misconceptions, biases, and emotions, prejudices, etc. This concept is becoming increasingly recognized and being addressed by certain minorities who see that they are being held back by the use of outdated expressions. For example, *chairman* conveys a subliminal message that only men act in managerial capacities, whereas *chairperson,* does not.

By verbally expressing certain thoughts, we expose ourselves to another's response, which can be negative and harmful. This does not mean that we must altogether avoid expressing our thoughts, many of which help us and others to learn and grow and which elicit valuable responses. Rather, we should be aware of the risk in certain situations for which another's negativity can harmfully sway us over the threshold. As was stated earlier in this chapter, under "Advice to Beginners," beginning students of T'ai Chi Ch'uan are enthusiastic but have a shaky foothold in a discipline requiring much dedication, patience, and ability to withstand discouragement. Because of this susceptibility, beginners should be wary of discussing or exhibiting what they have learned to others; another's scorn for something not understood can easily discourage a beginner to the point of not continuing.

Whenever embarking on some new task, either at odds with establishment thinking (such as a self-healing program) or involving difficulty and discouragement (such as a weight-loss diet), it is important to be very mindful to be reserved about expressing this resolve. While many will be supportive, others, without realizing their impact, might say things such as, "They say that breakfast is the most important meal of the day; going without a substantial breakfast has serious health consequences."

Even if we are prepared for such negativity, it nevertheless has a subliminal effect on our resolve. Or, if we are not treading a beaten path, it amplifies any vestige of self-doubt we may have. Alice Holtman, with whom I studied meditation and healing, often said, "If you have a spiritual question, don't ask others' opinions. Rather, go into meditation. Any question you have will be resolved in three days *at the very most.*"

Finally, we must observe the implications of the words that we think and say, and try to eliminate those that have a negative or limiting effect. In the words of Alice Holtman, "The subconscious mind is like a slave. It will do whatever you tell it. That is how hypnosis works. We must not tell our subconscious anything that will sabotage our progress."

It is crucial that the limitations and pitfalls of language not only be understood but be counterbalanced through meditation, during which experiencing occurs directly, without the use of language.

Images

Images are frequently used in T'ai Chi Ch'uan as well as many other disciplines that have a strong mental aspect. The names of the movements refer vividly to scenes in nature or to other familiar things. For example the move "Cloud Hands" conjures up an image of billowy clouds drifting by and the morning mist rising. Cheng Man-ch'ing emphasized imagining the air to have the consistency of water when doing the form. In the sword form it is of value to imagine a continuation of the movement far beyond that which could ever be reached by the physical sword.

As valuable as these and other similar images are, at a certain point they are superseded by experiencing the essence of the movement or concept. Images are a means of achieving a certain experience and should not become limiting.

Critical Evaluation of Ideas

While we depend to a great extent on others for knowledge, we all know that blind acceptance of the statements of others leads to all manner of unpleasant consequences. Therefore, it is necessary to have clear-cut criteria by which we may safely evaluate the statements and opinions of others.

The lowest level of evaluation is an acceptance of information based on the credentials of the person from whom the information originates. Of course this does not mean that we should not listen to others. That would be the other extreme. We must listen carefully and be totally open to new ideas or ideas that contradict what we have believed all of our lives. However, in trying radical ideas "on for size," we should not discard our prior conceptual framework prematurely.

Similarly, in discussions with others, we must utter as true only that which we have discovered from or verified by *our own experience.*

Learning From Books

When I started T'ai Chi Ch'uan in 1970, there were few books on the subject in English. I bought and read all of these. Presently, there are hundreds of books on T'ai Chi Ch'uan in English. Many of these books are of much value to all levels of practitioners. Books containing translations of the principles, as originally set down in the "T'ai Chi Classics," are especially worthwhile. Each practitioner should own at least one such book containing the words of the legendary masters.

Learning from a Videotape

At the present time, there are many videotapes of martial-arts forms and applications, and some of these videotapes are of much value if properly used. It is essential to keep in mind that a teaching videotape is of limited value unless used by (a) a practitioner with a strong foundation in the art being taught or (b) a beginner who also receives corrections directly from an experienced teacher.

For the experienced practitioner, videotapes make it possible not only to observe differing interpretations of forms already learned but, also, to acquire new forms with a substantial understanding. For the beginner whose failing memory after class is a problem, a teaching videotape can accelerate the rate at which new moves are learned.

One method of learning a form from a videotape is to repeatedly do the entire form or blocks of the form along with the videotape. However, this method is not efficient because there is insufficient opportunity to reinforce each movement. A better way is to refrain from doing the movements while watching the videotape. Rather, it is good to choose a small block of material, watch it a few times, and then stop the recorder (not on "pause," which can be disconcerting). Next, rewind the tape to the beginning of that block of material, to provide immediate reference if needed. Then, without any major physical action, visualize the sequence of movements as clearly as possible. Only after clear and complete visualization is achieved should the movements be attempted physically. If the visualization is still unclear or incomplete after a reasonable number of attempts, then replay that block of material.

At first it will seem extremely difficult to work this way. With persistence, however, it is possible to achieve a level of visualization so intense that the imagined movements are almost as vivid as those seen on a TV screen.

The dividends of the process of visualization are twofold: (1) By subduing the physical aspects of movement (e.g., balance, coordination, kinetic sense, timing), you can completely focus the mind on the details of the movement. (2) By cultivating the ability to visualize and mentally encompass complex details, you become increasingly able to observe and learn new movements quickly, especially in situations where it is not feasible to move while observing (e.g., dreams, the teacher showing movements while the class watches). In the realm of self-defense, the more you can observe the movements of the opponent, the greater the advantage achieved.

Learning From Dreams

Intense involvement in the study of T'ai Chi Ch'uan frequently evokes vivid dreams, from which new concepts are learned. These dreams should be taken seriously. They can be explained in various ways. One explanation is that these concepts are already subconsciously known but are revealed to the conscious mind through the dream. It is likely that the revelations of some dreams may be totally or partially of this nature. However, many people who study spiritual teachings eventually come to accept that, at times, revelatory information is being transmitted by *external* consciousness.

It is almost impossible to intensively study a Teaching that dates back to antiquity without also becoming attuned to consciousness who were or are similarly involved.

In my dreams I teach as often as I am taught. What I teach is frequently a revelation to me. In some dreams I give advice or administer healing to those with injuries. In other dreams I am given subtle corrections to my movements. Or, I am taught new movements, principles, and applications. In some cases I recognize those who are teaching me or to whom I am ministering. Some of these are in living human bodies. Others are those who are no longer in living human bodies.

For example, a few years ago my sister (who *is* alive) was attending a series of seminars on health and healing. She came to me in a dream and said, "The body will suffer great indignities without complaining because it does not want to be a pest. Therefore, we must be especially sensitive to harm we inflict on the body before the body tells us by our losing our state of health." I frequently quote these wise words to myself and to others.

In a dream I had shortly after Professor Cheng died, he watched over me as I did the "Preparation" movement of the form. After I stepped into the feet-parallel stance, he pointed out that I should then release residual tension in the insides of my thighs. When I awoke, I skeptically tried this movement. To my surprise, I found the correction to be absolutely valid. I never had any awareness of that unnecessary tension before the dream. Was it really Professor Cheng? I feel it was.

Hardly a week goes by that I do not have a revelatory dream.

When I was a beginning student, I used to have the following recurring T'ai Chi Ch'uan nightmare: I would be doing the form, and my arms would uncontrollably flail. I had this unpleasant dream dozens of times. In class one day, a senior student led us through the form very fast. Before, I had never done the form this fast. In my waking state, I now experienced a reminder of that awful but familiar feeling of the flailing arms. I then realized that my arms were too loosely connected to my body. I had *overdone* being relaxed. I then started to introduce a minute and subtle expansive tension to increase the connectedness of my arms to my body. Never again did I have that nightmare.

Taking Notes in Class

As a physics teacher, I sometimes admonish students to *stop taking notes and listen.* There are times when writing in class detracts from the learning experience. However, every now and then, a moment arrives when either the teacher's words or your own insights must be captured. It is then crucial that writing implements be within reach.

My experience is that T'ai Chi Ch'uan teachers do not mind note-taking when done within reason.

After class, the student should rewrite the notes in an expanded fashion. It is important that writing be done (a) in a bound book used solely for class notes and (b) soon enough that the thread of what was taught is not lost. The date of each entry should be included.

Keeping a Journal

Anyone involved in self-cultivation should spend some time every day writing down questions, insights, perceptions, and dreams. Daily writing produces a permanent record of your progress. The written record provides continuity to the learning process and reduces the probability that subtle insights will be lost. Moreover, because writing necessitates organization and clarity, it improves the mind.

At first, writing is quite difficult, but, as time progresses, your writing skill will improve noticeably. This improvement is a valuable fringe benefit.

It is important to keep a separate bound book of what is written. Moreover, the date should be recorded each time. Some people carry around and write on 3" X 5" index cards. Later they transfer what has been written to a more permanent journal.

Notes

1. Cheng Man-ch'ing, *T'ai Chi Ch'uan: A Simplified Method of Calisthenics for Health & Self-Defense,* pp. 1–2.

2. Robert W. Smith, *Chinese Boxing: Masters and Methods,* Kodansha International, Ltd., Tokyo, 1974, p. 51.

3. United States Department of Agriculture, *Composition of Foods,* U. S. Government Printing Office, Washington, DC, 1963, item 143.

4. Pa-Kua Chang is one of the three "internal" Chinese systems of self-defense (see Robert W. Smith, *Pa-Kua: Chinese Boxing for Fitness and Self-defense,* Kodansha International Ltd., Tokyo, Japan, 1967).

CHAPTER 9

Health, Healing, and Sexuality

Health, healing, and sexuality are so extensive that the treatment of each of these subjects could easily fill an entire book. Therefore, this chapter will leave much unsaid.

WHAT IS HEALTH?

Many people think that health is the absence of disease. However, a truly healthy person is not one who just happened not to get sick. Rather, true health also involves the mind. The mind must direct everything that affects the best interests of one's purpose in being alive and must take an active part in maintaining the body as an optimal dwelling place. T'ai Chi Ch'uan and other relevant teachings lead to a gradual accepting of responsibility and a corresponding ability to reverse or arrest adverse conditions.

HOW IS OPTIMAL HEALTH ATTAINED?

The inborn knowledge of the body is vast. Our cells know how to repair themselves without intervention. In most cases, only common-sense, hygiene, rest, and a justified faith in the ability of our body to restore its health are needed. However, there is a wealth of knowledge of healing, nutrition, digestion, beneficial and harmful effects of sunlight, effects of excesses, etc., available to us and of great benefit to know. Some of this knowledge is thousands of years old, and some is relatively recent.[1]

INJURIES

Learning from Injuries

Injuries are commonly regarded as setbacks and are not thought of as having any beneficial value. In fact, there is much that can be learned from an injury (as is true of all "loss"). First, the pain of an injury sensitizes the region involved and therefore increases our awareness of proper and improper alignment and body use. This awareness teaches us not only about the injured part but it improves our present and future use of healthy parts.

Next, actively participating in the healing process rather than blindly depending on medical or outside help provides an opportunity to increase our knowledge of healing and improve our ability to apply this knowledge. Last, we have the joy of witnessing the constructive aspect of nature operating within us and of knowing that we facilitated this wonderful process.

Pain

Pain is a mechanism that alerts us to that which can cut short our stay in the physical world. Suppressing pain rather than getting to the root of it only thwarts a beneficial mechanism. Interestingly, once the cause of the pain is addressed, the pain often subsides even if the trauma has not yet fully healed. While we should not seek pain, we should recognize its value and heed its call.

I have noticed that pain is sometimes experienced during the initial stages of healing. When I studied with Elaine Summers, she explained that this pain resulted from the "awakening" of nerves, which were traumatized and temporarily "asleep." This is an example of "good" pain.

Treating Injuries

Those who study martial arts become gradually aware that the same knowledge of bones, joints, tendons, muscles, nerves, and organs that can be used to do harm to one who attacks us, can be similarly used to prevent us from becoming harmed. Moreover, this complementary knowledge is also used to reverse the damage of an injury.

The concept of complementary knowledge is understood by the Chinese. In New York City's Chinatown, there is an herb shop whose window displays many remedies, such as ginseng roots, sea horses, and antlers. In addition, a collection of photographs of the proprietor of the shop is prominently displayed. These photographs show him in a variety of martial poses. Some poses are "empty handed," and the other poses are with different classical Chinese weapons. The implication is that the proprietor has a high-level knowledge of how to take you apart, and, therefore, he also has a correspondingly high level of knowledge of how to put you back together.

When I first began studying with Harvey Sober, a few of us would come early to class to do stretching or to practice. There was a young woman in the room who was not a classmate but was there practicing cartwheels. When she left, some of us became inspired to try doing cartwheels. Sober arrived, and one student, who was embarrassed at having been observed, immediately asked Sober whether cartwheels had any self-defense value. Sober replied, "Stand over there, and don't move" Then he distanced himself and did a cartwheel, kicking the student right over his eye. The kick would have just missed had the student remained stationary, as instructed. His face started to swell and change color. Sober said, "I told you not to move. Here, let me fix it." Sober's hands then proceeded to shape the student's face. Next, Sober held one hand near the injury for about a minute. The swelling and reddening were now visibly diminished. At this point, the student started to rub the injury with his hand. In frustration, Sober then said, "Now that you have ruined my work I have to do it again." Sober repeated the healing and said, "Don't touch it this time."

Next week, I came to class especially curious about the student's face. It was completely normal.

Ch'i

When a part of the body is injured, the skin, muscles, tendons, ligaments, blood vessels, nerves, and even the bones, glands, and organs may be traumatized to some degree. Western medicine believes in prompt application of ice to the traumatized area. The following is an explanation of why ice has a therapeutic effect: An important part of the damage that occurs from an injury is to the nerves. The damaged nerves in the affected region send random impulses, some of which result in further damage to the already traumatized tissues, including the nerves themselves. Thus a vicious cycle begins. This cycle can be interrupted by cooling the traumatized region to the point where nerve impulses are reduced.

Even though ice does help to arrest the secondary trauma, it does not address the fact that an injury causes the normal flow of Ch'i to become disrupted. Ch'i must be reinstated to avoid a substantial delay or even a halt in healing. This is why it is essential to come into touch with the normal flow of Ch'i and know how to reestablish this normal flow if it is disrupted. While ice may not always be available, Ch'i is always available in any amount. My teacher, Professor Cheng, said, "Ch'i is unlimited. Take as much as you like—no one will ever accuse you of being greedy."

Except for broken bones or deep cuts, it is usually possible to completely reverse the injury in a matter of minutes by sending Ch'i to the region of trauma. I have found that it is most important to start immediately. The longer the application of Ch'i is delayed, the longer it takes to recover from the injury.

Dit Da Jow

Dit da jow (literally translated as "rice hit wine") is a preparation containing about a dozen traditional Chinese herbs steeped in rice wine and aged for six months or longer. The basic formula has many variations and may well incorporate herbal knowledge that originated in China almost 5,000 years ago. It is usually topically applied to the skin (through which it is absorbed) to treat injuries of muscles, tendons, ligaments, and bones. There are many people who swear that minor to moderately severe injuries recover almost immediately after dit da jow is applied. My experience has borne out the effectiveness of this amazing preparation.

Those interested in learning more about dit da jow are referred to two fascinating articles on the subject by Brian Gray.[2]

Broken Bones

A break in a bone can occur in a joint or between two joints. When the break occurs *between two joints,* there can be a discontinuity in the shape of the original structure of the bone as well as a discontinuity in the movement of the two severed parts. Moreover, any tendency toward movement is accompanied by severe pain because any movement is produced by the contraction of a muscle, which, in turn, is attached to the bone by a tendon.

When the break occurs *in the joint,* there may be a floating piece of bone that clings to the cartilage and surrounding tissue. Because there is no muscular attachment to the floating piece, there may be relatively little pain associated with movement. The danger is that the fragment can work its way into the cartilage and eventually cause a deterioration of the joint.

In the case of very fragile bones, such as those in elderly people or those suffering from osteoporosis, a fracture can be caused by such a small force that there is little trauma to the surrounding tissue. Consequently, little pain is experienced.

Whenever a broken bone is suspected, it is wise to get an x-ray. If the bone requires setting, it is essential that this be done promptly by a qualified person. If the bone is broken, the most important requirement is immobilization. Once the knitting process begins, any relative movement of the two parts is detrimental.

The healing process begins with a "blood scab," which forms during the first week. The next stage is the deposition of bone. It normally takes about six to eight weeks before the broken bone reaches a substantial recovery of strength. However, the trauma to the surrounding tissues may take much longer to heal.

The healing process is accelerated by sending Ch'i to the traumatized area, with a special concentration of the Ch'i into the marrow of the bones.[3] Additionally, calcium supplements are considered to be beneficial.

Bruises

The immediate application of Ch'i is by far the most effective remedy. The Ch'i can be sent either externally, by sending it with one's hand, or internally, by mentally sending it directly to the problem area.

Sprains

A sprain is a stretched ligament. As with bruises, Ch'i should be applied to a sprain immediately. For those who are unable to treat themselves with Ch'i, the next best remedy is to chafe the traumatized region for about twenty minutes. Physical manipulation should be avoided if a fractured bone is suspected. Then, the remedy of choice would be the prompt application of ice and subsequent professional attention.

Tendonitis

Tendons are connective tissue connecting bone with muscle. When repeated stress is placed on tendons, they can become very painful. The most important factor is the early recognition of the symptoms and the immediate cessation of the offending activity.

The best treatment for tendonitis is rest and gentle massage. Controlled, stress-free movement is also helpful.

Cuts

Cleanliness is probably the most important consideration. I have found that flushing the wound with clean water makes disinfectants unnecessary. Bandaging a cut prevents entry of dirt, decreases the probability of further trauma, and keeps the wound from drying out.

Scrapes

The problem with a scrape is that a relatively large surface area of protective skin is absent. The formation of a scab, while temporarily protective, ultimately prolongs healing time. The dry, stiff scab tends to crack or be torn off. I have found that it is best to first remove any embedded dirt with water and a soft, clean toothbrush. Next, I apply clean saliva and a bandage. The bandage insures that the wound is kept clean and moist, so that a scab does not form.

Infections

I have found that treating local infections with hot water is very effective. I work up to the highest temperature that will not cause any scalding or injury. Momentarily elevating the temperature of the infected region does two things: (1) the higher temperature seems to lower the ability of the bacteria to multiply, and (2) the higher temperature stimulates the flow of blood to the area. The blood brings oxygen and nutrients and washes away toxins.

Massage

Massage has a number of effects. An obvious effect is to stimulate the circulation of blood to an area of the body, thereby facilitating the elimination of wastes and toxins and the absorption of oxygen and nutrients. Another effect is the stimulation of the flow of Ch'i. A less-frequently mentioned effect is that of sensitizing the massaged area so that, after the massage, your awareness of how that part is used becomes increased. Lastly, massage brings to our awareness areas that are in trouble but were insufficiently painful to notice. These last two benefits are educational. The recipient of massage that is done correctly and at the right time not only benefits from an immediate improvement in the health of the tissues involved but learns and later remembers something about those tissues.

Self-massage has the advantage that one is self-reliant and can therefore remedy a problem immediately rather than waiting for another to do the massage. Moreover, with self-massage, there is optimal feedback, and you know just the right degree of pressure, etc.

One disadvantage of self-massage is that it is difficult to reach all parts of the body. However, when I studied Kinetic Awareness with Elaine Summers, she taught me how to massage every part of my body using rubber balls of different sizes. While Summers' teaching extended far beyond simple massage, the massage aspect can be described as follows: Let us say that you need to massage a region between the shoulder blades. Lie on the floor and place a ball under the spot in question. The best type of ball is one that is air-filled rubber—not plastic. Such balls are obtained in toy stores and have familiar red, white, and blue stripes and other designs involving stars and animals. Spongy balls can also be used. Keep in mind that the smaller and harder the ball, the more penetrating it will be.

Next, relax completely for a while, and then try to move the part that is in contact with the ball. By rolling on the ball a small amount, the point of contact can be varied.

After a while or, if pain or discomfort dictates, roll off the ball and rest for a period of time. This rest is *very important* in order to allow the blood to flush the involved muscles and to allow the muscles to recover from their excursion into an unaccustomed lengthening. Getting up too soon can cause a serious muscular spasm.

Using a ball for self-massage in the above manner has the advantage that it takes very little or no effort, and the body can completely relax. It also has the advantage that the ball can penetrate much more deeply than is possible by using the hands.

Rubs

Rubs are self-massages to stimulate the natural flow of Ch'i to the organs or to the extremities. These rubs were taught to me by Cheng Man-ch'ing. Each rub has an optimal number of repetitions, as indicated (e.g., 49X). Some of the rubs are done either 49 or 108 times. Note that twice 49 is 98, *not* 108.

1. **Kidneys.** 49 (or 108) times. Place the backs of the wrists against the kidney area at the base of the ribs. Both wrists are brought downward and inward towards the coccyx, and then they are brought back upward. This down-and-up movement is counted as one cycle.

2. **Head.** 36 times. Using the fingers and palms of both hands with moderate pressure, massage the head upward, starting at the base of the hair and ending up at the crown of the head. The path should be varied so that all areas of the scalp receive equal benefit. This rub helps to bring Ch'i and blood to the brain and scalp and is especially beneficial to the hair follicles. I am convinced that doing this rub has arrested and even somewhat reversed my own balding.

   I observed Professor Cheng doing this rub on many occasions. He had a full head of hair when he was in his seventies.

3. **Eyes.** 36 times. Place the forefingers against the forehead over the eyebrows. Starting at the outside corner of each eye, rub the knuckle of each thumb inward along the upper bony ridge of the eye socket and then outward along the lower ridge. This circular movement should be done in a continuous manner.

4. **Abdomen.** 49 (or 108) times. Place the right hand, palm down, with the thumb against the right side of the abdomen at waist level. The hand is then moved to the left. Next, the hand rotates so that the palm faces upward. At the same time, the tips of the fingers gently press against the left side of the abdomen. Next, the hand is drawn back to the right, palm up, with the outer edge of the hand against the lower abdomen at a level just above the pubic bone. Finally, the hand is rotated to a palm-down orientation. At the same time, the heel of the hand gently presses against the right side of the abdomen. The circular motion just described is repeated forty-nine (or 108) times.

While Cheng did not state this, the above motion of the hand follows the natural motion of the contents of the intestinal tract during digestion: upward through the ascending colon (right side), across through the transverse colon, and downward through the descending colon (left side). The following anecdote should illustrate the value of the above rub for an acute condition: One day, about a year after I had started studying T'ai Chi Ch'uan, I suffered from extreme abdominal cramps after eating an indigestible item of food. It was as though my upper intestines were saying, "Get this poison out of here." At the same time, my lower intestines seemed to say, "Don't give that poison to us." In my agony resulting from this impasse, it occurred to me to try the abdominal rub. The speed with which the cramps disappeared was impressive. Elaine Summers taught me that therapeutic massage is best done when the musculature is relaxed. This concept is especially true of abdominal massage, for which it is necessary to penetrate to the organs beneath the musculature. Therefore, for the above acute condition, the abdominal massage was done while lying on my back, with my knees up. However, when the abdominal rub is done for building Ch'i, then you can remain standing.

5. **Feet.** 49 (or 108) times. Place the palm of one hand against the arch of the opposite foot, with the fingers pointed toward the front of the foot. Rub towards the front of the foot until the heel of the hand reaches the ball of the foot. The hand is then lightly drawn back to the starting position. This cycle is repeated forty-nine (or 108) times.

6. **Hands.** 21 times. Grasp the thumb heel of the left hand between the thumb and the first two fingers of the right hand, palm down. Using uniform pressure, draw the right hand toward the tip of the thumb of the left hand, as though squeezing the blood into the tip of that thumb. Then repeat with the index finger and then with the middle finger of the left hand. Next, grasp the tip of the fourth finger of the left hand between the thumb and the first two fingers of the right hand, palm up. Using uniform pressure, draw the right hand toward the heel of the left hand, as though squeezing the blood into the base of that finger. Then repeat on the last finger. This cycle is repeated twenty-one times. Then repeat the entire series on the other hand.

VISION

Vision defects, such as myopia (near-sightedness) can result from improper use of the eyes. Additionally, headaches can result from tension in the area of the eyes. Correct practice of T'ai Chi Ch'uan improves vision from the standpoints of both health and self-defense. During practice, the eyes are allowed to liquefy and relax. At the same time, more visual information can be processed because the eyes do not fixate on any particular object.

Palming

While not part of T'ai Chi Ch'uan, palming is considered to be one of the most beneficial therapies for the eyes. The procedure is to rub your hands together to warm them and energize them with Ch'i. Next cup your hands over your eyes for a period of about five minutes. The object is to liquefy the eyes and to experience the darkness and warmth. The eyes can be either completely or partially closed—whichever is more comfortable.

Palming should not end by suddenly opening the eyes. Instead, the hands are slowly removed, allowing the relaxed, closed eyes to receive light without processing any images. After a while, the eyes are slowly opened. The idea is to teach the eyes to function while retaining the state of relaxation that was experienced in darkness.

Our eyes slavishly do our bidding hour after hour. They are forced to receive light in a myriad of patterns that are continually processed by our nervous system. Because of electric lighting, this processing is extended long past the setting of the sun. Moreover, the muscles of our eyes are expected to focus on and follow events for extended periods of time. It is therefore extremely important that some rest be given to the eyes—if only for a few minutes.

FEET

Next to our stomachs, feet are possibly the most misunderstood and abused parts of our body. Because the feet are located at the lowest point, they bear the full body weight. Moreover, since they are used for standing and locomotion, they are seldom given a chance to rest. Additionally, footwear, which is necessary to protect our feet from weather, broken glass, and dirt, has evolved into a structure that debilitates and atrophies the muscles of the feet and prevents adequate ventilation. Finally, we anesthetize ourselves to the messages sent from our feet to our minds. In short, for many people, feet are essentially lifeless appendages, cut off from any awareness of correct function or care.

Arches

The arch of the foot is one of the three "shock absorbers" of the body. The other two are the knees and the spinal curves. The shock absorbing action of the knees is obvious. As stated before, if the spine were to consist of vertebrae stacked one upon another along a straight line rather than along their familiar curved line, a sudden mechanical shock would tend to have a harmful compressing effect. Rather, the curves of the spine result in a flexing action that absorbs shocks. Similarly, when the arch of the foot is supported with built-in arch supports, the arch loses its ability to flex, and every step sends a shock through the entire body.

It is a widespread misconception that shoes without arch supports will cause "fallen arches." How did this idea originate? The likely answer is as follows: All footwear is detrimental in proportion to the degree that it prohibits movement of the foot. Stiff shoes do not allow use of the muscles of the feet, and, consequently, these muscles atrophy. In particular, the muscles associated with the bones of the arch atrophy, and the arch collapses. Of course, this collapse is because of stiff footwear rather than a lack of support. All that the arch support of a stiff shoe does is limit the degree to which the arches collapse while the shoe is on the foot. However, if the stiff footwear were never worn, the arch would remain functional. Furthermore, the presence of an arch support, which presses upward against the arch of the foot when the shoe is worn, trains the foot to expect such pressure and predisposes that foot to fallen arches.

It is especially sad when young children, who are just learning to walk are fitted with slippery, stiff shoes. At that age, the arch has not yet formed, and, because of the shoes, it probably never will. Such stiff footwear prevents the child from sitting in the manner that all children naturally do, with their buttocks on or between their heels. Instead, the pressure of the ridge at the back of the shoe painfully cuts into the Achilles tendon, and, consequently, the child adjusts his or her feet to point outward, with the inside of the ankle against the floor. This alignment places severe torsional strain on the ligaments of the knee, and can cause permanent injury. Not all people who work with children are aware that this toe-out sitting is harmful. If an aware adult prevents the child from sitting with toes out, the child is then saved from injury but deprived of what would be, without shoes, a highly beneficial sitting position. Sitting on the floor is so beneficial because, among other things, it trains youngsters to experience correct spinal alignment. In cultures where children are not given chairs with backs and are encouraged to sit on the floor with bare feet, not only is posture better but also vision and rate of learning.

Four Reasons Why Fallen Arches are Harmful

1. The shock-absorbing function of the arch is lost, as mentioned above.

2. When the arch collapses, the ankle is moved inward, away from the center of the foot. Under the pressure of the full body weight, the ankle is much more vulnerable to becoming sprained when there is an unexpected unevenness in the ground. This vulnerability is multiplied by a leverage factor proportional to the height of the built-up heel of the shoe (more about heels later).

3. Collapsing the arch produces an excessive pressure on the first metatarsal. This leads to corns, calluses, and bunions.

4. Collapsing the arch tends to cause the knee to turn inward and greatly increases the vulnerability to a sprained knee ligament or worse.

Rehabilitation of Fallen Arches

There are two categories of flat feet:

1. **Congenital.** The structures have formed abnormally because of genetic rather than environmental factors. For congenital flat feet, it is best not to tamper but to recognize that attempting to alter this condition—especially through use of arch supports—is fruitless at best and may even be even harmful.

2. **Functional.** The feet have become flat through wrong use or because of an incorrect idea of how the feet should be used.

The following is the method I was taught by Elaine Summers to determine whether a student of mine has congenital or functional flat feet: I ask students to stand with bare feet, parallel, about one-half shoulder width apart. Then they bend their knees and spread the knees apart as much as possible without lifting the first metatarsal off the floor. Next, the knees are straightened while keeping them spread apart. Any improvement in the alignment of the arch is an indication that the problem is functional rather than congenital. The inability of a person to bend and straighten, as just outlined, is still not proof that the flat feet are congenital. It may be that some muscles have become so foreshortened and others so weak that the movement takes more strength than the student presently has. If I see that the problem stems from another part of the body such as the inner thighs, I suggest an exercise for that. If another cause is ruled out, I ask the student to attempt the bending, spreading, and straightening as a daily exercise for one week, after which a reassessment is made.

A number of reactions occur. The most common reaction is that after the bending and straightening, the student will say, "This feels very unnatural. I can't walk this way!" My reply is that any change from a habitual pattern of many years always feels "unnatural." I emphasize that it is not necessary to go the full way but to reverse the malalignment slowly. Just an awareness on the part of students that they are collapsing the arch and an attempt to relieve this collapse is a good start.

The second most common reaction is that students become immediately aware that their fallen arches are self-imposed, and they correct them from that point on.

Over the past decade I have given corrections to hundreds of students with flat feet. A large proportion of these students have reversed the problem in a few weeks. Others are, in my view, capable of reversing the problem, but they revert back to their old habits. However, all of those who reverted back were able to alter their alignment for a period of time, indicating that their fallen arches were functional. Although I do not completely reject the idea that congenital flat-footedness exists, I have not seen one case of it, and I suspect that it is either rare or essentially nonexistent.

A useful idea, as stated before but bears repeating, is to think of the foot as a tripod, with the three points being the first metatarsal, the last metatarsal, and the heel.

Effect of Excessive Weight

I have observed that those who are substantially overweight have a much more difficult time reversing flat feet. There is a limit to the ability of the muscles of the foot to maintain a proper arch under excessive pressure. Therefore, if any corrections are to be taken seriously, weight loss must come first.

Foot Exercises

The kind of shoes that encase the modern, Western foot prevent any sort of normal muscular movement. Consequently, the muscles of such a foot tend to become atrophied, and the foot then loses much of its strength and flexibility. People whose hands have become non-functional learn to use their feet to write, pick up the telephone, and turn doorknobs. This dexterity indicates the extent to which the average foot falls short of fulfilling its potential flexibility. While learning to write with one's feet is hardly advisable for the average person, it is of value to spend a few minutes a day in exercising the feet. One of the best exercises for the muscles and tendons of the feet is to make a fist with the foot. This action should be done very cautiously, to avoid muscle spasms. As the muscles of the feet regain their tone, it will be possible to make a tight fist with the foot, similar to that which can be formed with a hand. This exercise strengthens the arch and lengthens the tendons that lift the toes. Because most shoes have such rigid soles, the feet seldom have a chance to clench. However, the shoes can bend upward and are often fixed in this position because of the built-up heels. Thus the tendons that lift the toes become foreshortened in the feet of most people to the extent that even when the foot is in the relaxed state, the outlines of these foreshortened tendons are visible on the top of the foot. Making a fist with the foot is the best way to reverse this imbalance. The best time to exercise the feet is just after washing them, when the increased blood circulation and warmth reduces the tendency of the muscles to undergo spasm. Another good time to exercise the feet is just after awakening but before putting any weight on the feet. The likelihood of a spasm of the foot muscles will be greatly reduced as the muscles regain their tone and flexibility.

FOOTWEAR

Heels on Shoes

Built-up heels do not do the feet any good. Firstly, they foreshorten the Achilles tendon, which, in most people, is so short that it does not need any further shortening. Secondly, they shift the pressure, from being more uniformly distributed over the sole of the foot, to being mainly concentrated on the metatarsals. This pressure leads to calluses, corns, and bunions. Lastly, the heels cause the center of mass of the person to shift forward. To compensate, the person must lean backward, arching the lower back, leading to lower-back problems. Lastly, the heel produces leverage that increases the vulnerability of an improperly aligned ankle.

Select footwear that is designed from the very beginning with the functioning of the feet foremost. It may surprise you to know that this problem was solved quite a few thousands of years ago by the primitive peoples of the world who brought the art of footwear design to its highest level. George M. White describes dozens of designs of "primitive" footwear.[4]

Wearing-Down of Heels

It is my belief that the outer edges of heels tend to wear down mostly because people who walk with their feet angled out tend to scuff that part of the shoe on the ground. Such wear patterns do not necessarily represent the pressure distribution on the sole of the foot, as is commonly believed.

Ideal Footwear

Footwear worn by people who must walk on pavement, etc. should have the following qualities:

1. The footwear should be flexible, soft, and, at the same time, have a sole thick and be resilient enough to cushion the foot from sharp objects and mechanical shock. That is, the foot must not be restricted in its muscular action but must also be protected.

2. The footwear should have neither a raised heel nor arch. The heel should not be lower either.

3. The footwear should breathe. Thus, except possibly for the outer soles, artificial substances such as plastic are ruled out.

4. The footwear must be aesthetically pleasing. Of course, styles have evolved that demonstrate a perverted sense of aesthetics that is not easy to reverse. However, the Native American footwear is so simple and practical that most people appreciate its beauty. I have crafted and worn various adaptations of Ute Indian footwear for more than a decade. By comparison, conventional footwear would feel like vises on my feet. The skin on my feet is as smooth as that of a baby, and I can stand on my feet a full day without the slightest fatigue or discomfort.

Short of making your own shoes, the best solution is to buy Chinese "kung-fu slippers." For everyday wear, these shoes are optimal and inexpensive. They can be obtained at Oriental clothing or variety stores.

An Anecdote. A few years ago, I wanted to purchase a pair of running shoes. I went to a large store that sold running shoes exclusively, in the hope that a large store might stock running shoes of approximately my EEEE width. There was one pair of size EEE, which would have been satisfactory were it not for a huge built-in arch support. I knew that I would never be able to wear such a shoe. Out of desperation I said to the salesman, "I am going to try to make my own running shoes." The salesman replied, "You can make shoes?" When I told him that I made the footwear that I was wearing, he said "I would be very interested to see any running shoes you make. Please come back and show them to me."

I made a pair of shoes using a porous type of leather into which I punched holes at regular intervals. I used a thick spongy crepe for soles and glued to that a rubber sole with large, springy saw-tooth ridges. (I have since run many miles in these shoes, and they function beautifully.)

When I returned to the store, the salesman was very interested and called the other salesman to see what I had made. They were impressed with the lightness of the shoes, the soles, and the fit. However, one salesman suddenly remarked, "These shoes have no support!" By this characterization he meant that there were no built-in arch supports. This situation was ironic because the main reason I went to the trouble of making my own running shoes was to eliminate the arch supports. However, another salesman said that he had just finished reading an article about African runners who win races without wearing any shoes—let alone arch supports. He added that the article mentioned that such supports may hamper the natural spring-like motion of the arch of the foot. I left the store happy that the truth about arches and their support is slowly emerging.

NUTRITION

T'ai Chi Ch'uan and Optimal Body Weight

It is sometimes said that those who study T'ai Chi Ch'uan lose body weight if they are overweight and gain if they are underweight. It is doubtful that there is any truth to this generalization. The incidence of "overweight" or "underweight" practitioners seems to parallel that of non-practitioners. If anything, there may even be a tendency for practitioners to gain weight because they become so relaxed and efficient. Perhaps the weight loss occurs for practitioners who engage more in weapons or fighting practice, which are more physically demanding.

Is the tendency of T'ai Chi Ch'uan practitioners to gain weight a disadvantage or an advantage? At first glance one would think that anything that might make it difficult to keep from losing weight must be a disadvantage. However, the tendency to gain weight results from an increased efficiency, which reduces the need to consume food. One should regard this increased efficiency as a blessing in disguise. Many health problems result from overeating. The less food we take in, the smaller the amount of poisons we ingest, the more efficiently we digest and absorb essential nutrients, and the less we are poisoned by the toxins from the decomposition of food in our gut by the action of bacteria and yeast.

SEXUALITY

The sexual organs of many males are among the most misused parts of the body. (The other two most misused parts of the body are the stomach and the feet.) Part of the reason for this sexual misuse is a currently prevailing openness toward and overemphasis on sex, which is an overreaction to a prior attitude of shame and denial of sex. Another factor is the ease, reliability, and availability of contraceptives. The belief of most males is, "The more sex, the better," and many people even feel that no form of sex between consenting adults is harmful. The sexual organs serve the biological function of reproduction. Just because the use of these organs results in a high degree of pleasure does not necessarily mean that that use is always beneficial to the individual to whom those organs belong. To be propagated, a particular biological feature of an organism need only insure that the organism live long enough to successfully reproduce. In nature there are examples of organisms that sacrifice their very lives to reproduce: the male preying mantis, Pacific-coast salmon, and many varieties of spiders.

The fact that humans can engage in the sexual act without guilt or conception has removed the only ostensible barriers to the male achieving frequent ejaculations. However, the less obvious effect of this frequency has the following serious consequences: The male ejaculate contains nutrients that are expelled, and these nutrients are removed from the blood, organs, and nervous system of the body at their expense. Therefore, achieving frequent ejaculations can adversely affect the physical and mental functioning of males. Moreover, spiritual energy is squandered when the sexual act—or any other act, for that matter—is carried to excess.

At the same time, sexual activity need not be avoided. Repressing it causes an expenditure of mental energy. The sexual act in moderation and with the correct mental attitude is a boost to the physical, mental, and spiritual aspects. Spiritual growth is cultivated when the main emphasis in the sexual act is on love rather than on the pleasure of the sexual organs, per se, or on possessing one's partner.

Taoist Sexual Practices

The overuse of the male sexual function stems not so much from engaging in the sexual act, per se, but rather from the ejaculation of semen. The idea that one can have a truly satisfying act of sexual intercourse without an ejaculation is totally foreign to the vast majority of men. However, not only is it possible to be totally satisfied without an ejaculation, it is also possible to achieve an intense orgasm without ejaculation. Therefore, once the ability to engage in sexual intercourse without ejaculation is acquired, sexual intercourse can be engaged in as frequently as desired without ill effect and, more likely, with substantial benefit.[5]

Learning to subdue the ejaculation is accomplished as follows: Shortly before ejaculation, there is a point where the sexual arousal increases but then momentarily subsides. When this subsiding is experienced, intercourse should be suspended. After a few minutes of rest, one can resume intercourse. At first, there will be a feeling of frustration because one is accustomed to a release of sexual tension that is sudden and intense rather than subtle and gradual. However, after a few times of experiencing the subtle version with its consequent feeling of energy, spirituality, and well-being, one will routinely avoid an ejaculation until it is absolutely necessary. Moreover, with practice, each successive build-up of sexual tension will culminate in an increasingly intense climax. These climaxes will eventually become at least as intense as those involving an ejaculation.

One way of preventing an unwanted ejaculation is to squeeze the anal sphincter when an ejaculation is imminent.[6] This and many other valuable techniques are fully described in the reference just cited.

The Chinese claim that the non-ejaculated semen is reabsorbed and turned into Ch'i. Whether or not this claim is literally true, engaging in sexual intercourse culminating in an orgasm without ejaculation heightens the flow of Ch'i. Additionally, when semen is not squandered, the mind will become increasingly clear.

Of course, every so often, an ejaculation will naturally occur, and the "dry" orgasm will be bypassed.

Ginseng

Ginseng root is widely known for its ability to reverse impotence. Taking ginseng for this effect must be done cautiously. Taking ginseng and then overindulging in sexual activity is like giving fertilizer to a faltering plant, thereby causing it to flower and then die. If ginseng is used, sexual activity must be subdued over a period of time until the system is rejuvenated.

Sex Fast

The vicious cycle of overuse can be broken with a sex fast. The person on a sex fast must abstain from all aspects of sex, both physical and mental. The sexual organs should not be stimulated in any manner, and the mind must remain far from any sexually stimulating thoughts. Spiced foods, highly salted foods, and foods containing monosodium glutamate or mustard are sexually stimulating (because of their irritation to the urinary tract) and must be avoided.

It is beneficial to continue such a fast for as long as a month. The sex fast is broken in a similar way as a food fast; that is, overindulgence is avoided. To jump back to overuse is probably worse than having never fasted in the first place.

Sleep

Naps

When I was a college student, there were times when I would work on an assignment so late into the night that it was completed only a few hours before the time to awaken for the next day's classes. My idea at the time was that it was better to stay up all night than to sleep for only a few hours. I based this idea on the fact that after awakening from such a short "night's" sleep I would feel awful for the whole day. I erroneously assumed that this feeling was from the sleep I got rather than the sleep I did not get.

As time went on it began to dawn on me that I really was worse off with no sleep than with a few hours sleep. Later, as a graduate student in physics (a demanding discipline) and as a physics instructor, there were many times when I was so exhausted that I literally would find an inconspicuous spot on the floor of an unused classroom and take a short nap. At first I was amazed to find that not only would I fall asleep in a short time but that sleeping for just a few minutes really refreshed me.

Over the years, I have improved steadily in my ability to fall into a deep sleep very quickly and to feel almost totally recharged after awakening a few minutes later. Presently, there is a rug-covered lab table in the back of my physics classroom, upon which I have taken hundreds of naps ranging in time from four or five minutes to a few hours. Every now and then, five minutes before the start of class, as my students are beginning to enter the classroom, I take a nap lasting a few minutes. I fall deeply asleep almost immediately and awaken feeling relaxed and invigorated. People who hear this are inclined to say, "I wish I could do that, but I know that I would never fall asleep under those conditions." My reply is that just lying down without sleeping will produce almost the same benefit. Moreover, with practice, you will learn to fall asleep in a shorter and shorter time.

There are three things that are good to know about naps. (1) In addition to the normal clothing, a blanket or the equivalent is important—especially over the trunk of the body. The internal organs need this extra warmth during a period of quiescence. (2) Removal of street footwear is important. Aside from the fact that the ventilation of the feet is of benefit, the removal of the footwear facilitates the mental transition from wakefulness to restfulness. (3) It is important not to worry about whether or not there may be a problem in arising refreshed but to trust that the body will benefit from the nap, no matter how short.

It is now known that it is even possible to fall asleep for a fraction of a second, and experiments on sleep have studied this *microsleep.*[7] In fact, it is thought that cases of people who have allegedly gone for extended periods of time without sleep have done so only because they actually did sleep for a fraction of a second at a time, and the total time spent in microsleep became significant.

Let us enumerate some of the benefits of a nap:

1. A nap is restful to the muscles of the eyes and the retina itself. Just think of how long the eyes are forced to remain open (except for short blinks) without rest from bright light. Moreover, the muscles of the eyes must continuously work, both to focus the eyes and direct the line of sight. A few minutes of rest and darkness are very important (see the discussion of palming in the section on vision earlier in this chapter).

2. The axis of the spine must remain essentially upright for a number of hours during wakefulness and needs rest. The effect of gravity acting along the axis of the spine temporarily compresses the discs and correspondingly decreases the space for the nerves therein. Try accurately measuring your height in the morning, after a night's sleep. (Stand with your back against a wall and place a book with one edge touching the top of the head and the other edge against the wall. Then make a mark on the wall where the lower corner contacts it.) Next, wait until the end of the day, and measure your height again. You will probably find that

your height increases as much as one inch during a long night's sleep and decreases as much as an inch during the day. Lying down gives the discs a chance to decompress, whether or not actual sleep occurs.

3. Over the course of many hours of wakefulness, the mind takes on a mode of mechanical thinking, which tends to be dissipated by a nap. A short nap is very refreshing to the mind and is restful to the parts of the nervous system that process visual sense data. Such processing, when overdone, is at the expense of other important mental functions. It is common to awaken from a nap with a more objective slant on a problem than before the nap.

Sleep Amounts

The vast majority of people suffer from inadequate amounts of sleep. When sleep is required but postponed, regenerative processes are reduced and are inefficient. The result is that a larger total amount of sleep is then required to reverse the harmful effects of the deprivation. The best time to get sleep is when the need is felt. If you want to spend less time sleeping, sleep more frequently and more promptly.

It will be found that practicing T'ai Chi Ch'uan or Ch'i kung daily will reduce the amount of sleep you need by much more than the practice time.

Pillows

Whether or not you should sleep on a pillow depends upon your individual spinal curves and whether or not you sleep on your side, back, or front. Since many people sleep in a variety of positions during the course of each night, it becomes valuable to have a pillow the thickness of which is easily varied. A pillow loosely filled with buckwheat hulls (these can be cheaply obtained in a garden-supply store) is ideal.

In general, a pillow of the proper thickness should help the spine and the joints of the body to attain a centered and stress-free alignment similar to that of an ideal standing position.

Notes

1. See, for example, *Arnold De Vries, Therapeutic Fasting,* Chandler Book Co., Los Angeles, CA, 1963; Herbert M. Shelton, *Food Combining Made Easy,* Dr. Shelton's Health School, San Antonio, TX, 1972; and Gary Price Todd, M.D., *Nutrition, Health, & Disease,* Whitford Press, West Chester, PA, 1985.

2. "Liquid Gold or Fool's Potion?" *Inside Kung Fu,* Vol. 19, No. 7, July, 1992 and "Dit Da Jow: Making Kung-Fu's Liquid Gold," *Inside Kung Fu,* Vol. 19, No. 10, October, 1992.

3. Yang Jwing-Ming, *Muscle/Tendon Changing and Marrow/Brain Washing Chi Kung—The Secret of Youth,* Yang's Martial Arts Association, Jamaica Plain, MA, 1989.

4. George M. White, *Craft Manual of North American Indian Footwear,* available from George M. White, P.O. Box 365, Ronan, Montana 59864.

5. See Jolan Chang, *The Tao of Love and Sex,* E. P. Dutton, New York, NY, 1977.

6. Dr. Stephen T. Chang, *The Tao of Sexology,* Tao Publishing Co., San Fransisco, CA, 1986.

7. William C. Dement, *Some Must Watch While Some Must Sleep,* p. 12.

CHAPTER 10

Miscellaneous

MALE AND FEMALE PRACTITIONERS

In certain disciplines, some people have an advantage over those of the opposite sex. Over the years that I have studied and taught T'ai Chi Ch'uan, I have observed that, except for individual differences, men and women make essentially equal progress on all levels.

ART AND T'AI CHI CH'UAN

Art is a spatial and/or temporal sequence of events, often in abstract representation, which involves a seemingly discordant, chaotic, or haphazard subject and resolves that chaos into harmony and balance using the highest level of creative intelligence. Familiar examples of art are music, painting, theater, cinema, and literature.

The most primitive forms of fine art are drawings that are highly representational (such as those found on cave walls, depicting a hunter and animals). However, even these drawings are abstract in the sense that they are really a wall and paint forming some sort of pattern. Modern art is much more abstract, and it is much harder to associate the patterns on canvas with events in the physical world. In fact, at some point it becomes unnecessary and even detracting to attempt this association.

The more primitive types of music contain words that refer to worldly events in an abstract but definitive manner. The rhythms simulate patterns of fetal and maternal heartbeats while in the womb. The beat corresponds to patterns of physical movement such as walking or running. The pitches and their combinations refer to the formants present in the human voice. The words *harmony, discord,* and *resolution* are used to refer to musical events because the main activity in musical composition is to make excursions away from harmony to discord and back to harmony. Conflict is created and then harmoniously resolved. That is why sound produced by a cat walking on the keyboard of a piano is not music although this sequence of sounds can be transformed into music by a genius. A transformation of this sort is exemplified by Domenico Scarlatti's *Cat's Fugue,* which is "...so called because the theme consists of wide and irregular skips in ascending motion, such as might be (and possibly were) produced by a cat walking on the keyboard."[1] Similarly, a child's (or childish adult's) random splashes of paint on a surface cannot be considered to be art because there is no element of harmony or balance, let alone creative thought.

In theater, the trend these days is to cultivate conflict between the characters but not necessarily to resolve that conflict. This trend results from the ease with which unresolved conflict can be generated and the fact that audiences no longer have the span of attention or intellectual capacity to follow a complex plot to its harmonious conclusion. Rather, many people are satisfied with being momentarily dazzled and overcome with strong emotion—even if this emotion is anger or fear. Because we live in a highly mechanized world, we have lost a sense of the beauty of nature. Moreover, many artists, playwrights, and composers are overwhelmed with the chaos they perceive, and they are unable to take the portrayal of this chaos to a higher creative level—its resolution.

The ecstatic joy felt when we experience great art is explained as follows: Each of us aspires to use our creative intelligence to increase the harmony of ourselves and of the world. This aspiration is the very reason that our consciousness have come into human bodies in the physical world. The physical world is characterized by "nature," in which harmony and conflict abound. We were placed here to experience nature and to learn how to use our creative intelligence to convert chaos and discord into harmony. When we succeed in our purpose, we are ecstatic. When we fail, we suffer.

Music involves a succession of auditory events analogous to daily events in the physical world. The difference between the harmony achieved in our daily lives and that in music is that, in our daily lives, we are seldom successful, whereas, in music, success has been ingeniously built in. When we follow the events in music with our minds, we experience a taste of the ecstasy that would be ours were we to apply our creative intelligence to the events in our lives to the degree displayed in the music.

People these days are so deprived of contact with undefiled nature and true spirituality, that there is a yearning, devoid of any sense of the *object* of this yearning. Because their daily lives lack creativity and meaning, people attempt to satisfy their yearning for upliftment by increasing the intensity of familiar but debasing experiences. For example, rather than become trained to listen to the subtleties in more creative and complex music such as that written by Bach, many people increase their experiencing of music by listening to a lower creative level of music but at a higher intensity level. In fact, the intensity levels to which some people have become accustomed are so great as to cause immediate and permanent hearing damage. Similarly, most food available in the supermarkets has not been grown in soil containing a full and balanced spectrum of trace minerals. Instead, this food is forced to grow by means of artificial methods. This manner of production requires adding such things as refined sugar, salt, vinegar, and spices to what

	Short Form	Long Form		Short Form	Long Form
Preparation	1	0	Separate Right Foot	1	1
Beginning	1	1	Separate Left Foot	1	1
Ward off with Left Hand	2	3	Turn and Strike with Sole	0	3
Ward off with Right Hand	3	5	Turn and Strike with Heel	1	0
Roll Back	4	7	Right Foot Kicks Upward	0	1
Press	4	7	Hit a Tiger at Left	0	1
Push	5	9	Hit a Tiger at Right	0	1
Single Whip	3	9	Right Foot Kicks Upward	0	1
Lift Hands	1	3	Strike Both Ears with Fists	0	1
Lean Forward	1	3	Left Foot Kicks Upward	0	1
The Crane Spreads its Wings	1	3	Parting the Horse's Mane (L)	0	1
Brush Knee Twist Step (L)	2	6	Parting the Horse's Mane (R)	0	1
Hands Playing the P'i P'a	1	2	Horizontal Single Whip	0	1
Brush Knee Twist Step (R)	1	2	Fair Lady Works at		
Chop with Fist	0	3	the Shuttles	4	4
Step Forward, Deflect Down-			Descending Single Whip	2	2
ward, Intercept, and Punch	2	6	Golden Cock Stands		
Apparent Close-Up	1	2	on One Leg (R)	1	1
Diagonal Single Whip	1	1	Golden Cock Stands		
Embrace the Tiger to			on One Leg (L)	1	1
Return to the Mountain	1	2	White Snake Puts Out Tongue	0	1
Looking at the Fist			Cross Palms	0	1
Under the Elbow	1	1	Turn and Cross Legs	0	1
Step Back to Repulse			Punch Opponent's		
the Monkey (R)	3	6	Pubic Region	0	1
Step Back to Repulse			Brush Knee and Punch Down	1	1
the Monkey (L)	2	4	Step Forward to the Seven Stars		
Diagonal Flying	1	2	of the Big Dipper	1	1
Needle at Sea Bottom	0	2	Step Back to Ride the Tiger	1	1
Fan Through Back	1	2	Turn the Body to		
Turn and Chop with Fist	0	2	Sweep the Lotus	1	1
Cloud Hands	3	9	Bend the Bow		
High Pat on Horse	0	2	to Shoot the Tiger	1	1
			Close Up	1	1
			Total	63	136

Table 10-1. *The Number of Occurrences of Postures of the Short and Long Forms.*

would otherwise be natural food. Some of these additives are highly concentrated nutrients in excess (refined sugar). Others, such as vinegar (5% acetic acid), are literally poisons (fatal dose: 13.5 ounces).[2] With physical as well as spiritual hunger, there is an indulgence to excess and or harm when the natural essence is either missing or unable to be sensed. So it is with every phase of human experience. It would seem that the increasing chaos and complexity of life would generate a corresponding creative impulse to resolve the chaos. Instead, the chaos is sought out, amplified, and sensationalized, which produces a vicious cycle.

The question naturally arises, how can this vicious cycle be reversed? Even if it cannot be reversed for the world in general, can it at least be mitigated for an individual by that individual? It is my belief that doing T'ai Chi Ch'uan is an excellent way to accomplish this reversal.

When we go to an unpopulated region with undefiled natural surroundings, such as trees, insects, birds, mountains, and streams, we have an opportunity to satisfy our yearning for contact with nature. Unfortunately, not many of us have much of an opportunity to commune with nature in this manner. However, we, ourselves, are microcosms of nature. That is, the laws of nature manifest within ourselves. Every thought we have and action we take has the potential to reveal nature to us and to reawaken our awe and experiencing of nature in a manner analogous to that evoked by contact with trees, insects, birds, etc. It is only for us to provide the mental conditions for our appreciation of nature within ourselves.

When we do T'ai Chi Ch'uan, we are actively using our minds to bring all of our body parts into harmony. When Ch'i is taken into account, it may be said that even the individual cells of our body come into harmony with each other. It is as though we are making music with our bodies in two senses: Our bodies are both the instrument through which the harmony is experienced and the subject of this harmonizing. The most beautiful aspect of T'ai Chi Ch'uan is that it requires absolutely no equipment or special clothing. It can be done alone and in a space as small as four feet square. As a result, it is a priceless possession—one that cannot be lost because it is totally within us.

DANCE AND T'AI CHI CH'UAN

It is common for people unacquainted with T'ai Chi Ch'uan to remark, "It looks just like ballet." What, if any, is the connection between dance and T'ai Chi Ch'uan? Of course, the obvious similarity is that both dance and T'ai Chi Ch'uan involve movements of the various parts of a human body in a well-defined manner. However, there is little additional similarity. In dance, the human body is used as an instrument to express the artistic ideas of the choreographer. Moreover, dance is usually performed for the benefit of an audience rather than primarily for the benefit of the dancers, themselves. Finally, the movements that the human body is required to make in dance are not necessarily physiologically correct or optimal, and sometimes they are injurious.

By contrast, the person doing T'ai Chi Ch'uan cares not what it looks like. If the movement is beautiful, it is because a human body, moving in accordance with principles of physiology and health, is beautiful to watch. The motive of the T'ai Chi Ch'uan practitioner is not to entertain others but to interconnect mind, body, and nature. T'ai Chi Ch'uan is not done to music but, rather, to an *inner* flow. The T'ai Chi Ch'uan movements were originated and refined by those who were highly knowledgeable about principles of movement, action, physiology, and health.

It must be mentioned that what has been said of dance is a generalization and does not hold for all types of dance. There are some dancers whose goals and methods are very much along the same lines as those of T'ai Chi Ch'uan, but these are not usually the dancers referred to by most people who regard T'ai Chi Ch'uan and dance as similar.

SCIENCE AND T'AI CHI CH'UAN

Science is the field of knowledge that describes, explains, and predicts natural phenomena. Scientific inquiry requires a high degree of skepticism, rigor, and training. Ironically, for most people, science is a form of religion; its conclusions are accepted without questioning. Most people stand in awe of the vast array of science's impressive accomplishments and are willing to accept everything that is couched in scientific phraseology. Such an unquestioning attitude is, of course, the very antithesis of a true scientific approach.

To predict dependably, science must limit its scope by eliminating from its field of view that which hampers analysis. Consequently, science has had much greater success with physical aspects of nature than with mental or experiential aspects.

Many who study spiritual disciplines regard the application of science to these disciplines to be of little value because scientists tend to explain spiritual experiences in a manner that negates the validity of these experiences. Unfortunately, the application of science to spiritual teachings is limited more by the spiritual development of the individual scientist involved than by an intrinsic attribute of science itself. As scientists become more spiritually evolved, scientific method will naturally begin to deal meaningfully with spiritual matters. Until then, the application of science to spiritual teachings will continue to be regarded as suspect by adepts at those teachings.

Nevertheless, science is quite useful when it comes to describing and understanding the physiological and movement aspects of T'ai Chi Ch'uan.

COMPARISON OF THE SHORT AND LONG FORMS

The term *long form* refers to the form taught by Yang Cheng-fu, containing 108 postures (more or less, depending on how the postures are counted). The term *short form* refers to an abridged version of the long form such as that originated by Cheng Man-ch'ing or, later, by others (see Table 10-1 for the number of occurrences of each posture in the short and long forms). It should be noted that, for each of these forms, there is some nonuniformity of the number of occurrences of certain movements from practitioner to practitioner.

Professor Cheng said that he found that one round of the long form, which he was taught by Yang Cheng-fu, took so long to complete that he tended to rush through the movements. Therefore, he reduced the repetitions of some movements or of sections of the form, eliminated a few movements, and slightly changed the order of the original movements. The only change in that order is his placement of "Descending Single Whip" and "Golden Cock Stands on one Leg" before the sequence involving "Separate Right Foot," "Separate Left Foot," and "Downward Punch." Repetitions of "Single Whip," "Cloud Hands," and "Brush Knee," which occur in the long form, also occur to a proportional degree in the short form. In general, the balance of the different types of movements is retained in the short form. Movements that were eliminated are "Chop with Fist," "Needle at Sea

Bottom," "High Pat on Horse," "Strike Tiger Right," "Strike Tiger Left," "Strike Both Ears with Fists," "Turn and Chop with Fist," "White Snake Puts Out Tongue," and "Parting the Wild Horse's Mane." While these omitted movements certainly are of value, they are not crucial. That is, enough exposure to the substance of T'ai Chi Ch'uan is present in the remaining movements of the short form.

The short form has the advantage that it is learned in a much shorter time than the long form but retains almost all of the basic types of movement of the long form. The short form allows the student to perfect the movements at an earlier stage of learning and to spend a greater proportion of time working on the principles rather than on learning new movements or sequences of movements.

Some say that a round of the short form takes so little time to do that many benefits are not achieved. As one who has practiced the long form for over a decade and the short form for over twenty-four years, I have observed that practitioners repeat the short form proportionally more than the long form, and, thus, the total amount of practice is equal.

Here I would like to tell a pertinent anecdote. As a student of the harpsichord, I was privileged to attend a series of small workshops with the late harpsichordist, Fernando Valenti. Valenti was a famous interpreter of the Scarlatti sonatas. Each of these five hundred fifty sonatas has two movements, both of which are always repeated. Valenti stated that, as a recording artist, he preferred to eliminate the repeats, thus enabling twice the number of sonatas to be recorded on one record album. He said, "If people want to hear the repeats, let them play back each sonata twice." Similarly, practitioners of the short form are free to repeat the whole form or parts thereof as often as desired.

After the short form is learned, it is then relatively easy to learn the long form in a very short time—the total learning effort being less this way. At some point, each practitioner should learn the long form. Once both forms are known, it will be discovered that there is no substantial advantage to the long form. In fact, any form is merely a vehicle for the transmission of the underlying concepts and knowledge.

VARIATIONS IN INTERPRETATION OF THE T'AI CHI CH'UAN MOVEMENTS
Straight or Bent Rear Leg?

A glance at pictures of Yang Cheng-fu will reveal that his rear leg was essentially straight in a 70-30 posture.[3] By contrast, Cheng Man-ch'ing emphasized a bent rear leg. Professor Cheng felt that releasing the knee and hip joint of the rear leg improved the alignment and relaxation of the pelvis and lower spine. Straightening the rear leg tends to make the body lean forward. The leaning is difficult to correct without either bending the rear leg or breaking the alignment of the lower back and pelvis.

Why Does the Rear Foot Pivot on the Heel Rather Than on the Toe?

In T'ai Chi Ch'uan, as practiced by those who pivot the rear foot, the force of the strike comes not from the rear leg (as in Karate) but from both legs. Straightening the rear leg or pivoting the rear foot on the ball actually prevents the body from turning and, therefore, from developing the maximum transfer of energy.

In Robert Smith's book, *Chinese Boxing,*[4] there are photographs taken in rapid sequence of Cheng Man-ch'ing defending against an attack. Cheng is seen to step toward the attacker with his right foot, push the attacker, and then follow through by sliding his rear foot forward, almost parallel to the right foot. Later in Smith's book,[5] there is a series of photographs of Wang Yen-Nien reacting in almost the same manner as Cheng.

Pivoting of the Empty Foot in "Brush Knee"

In doing the transition from "White Crane Spreads Wings" to "Brush Knee," practitioners from some Yang-style schools keep the forward (empty) foot pointed forward while turning the body to the right and then back. In his later years, Professor Cheng taught his students to *pivot* the forward foot on its ball in that movement so that the foot moves with and points in the same direction as the body.

Each of these variations has a distinct benefit. Not pivoting the foot requires the thigh joint of the forward leg to open, whereas pivoting the leg challenges the practitioner to connect the empty leg to the body, simultaneously keeping the optimal alignment. In defense of pivoting, there are many movements in the form that open the thigh joints, but there is essentially no other movement that gives the foot a chance to pivot in the same manner as does "Brush Knee." Of course, it is of value to practice both methods.

Straight or Bent Wrist?

See chapter 5 for a discussion of the different opinions about the alignment of the wrist.

Pre-Positioning the Rear Foot at the Beginning of a Movement Compared with Pivoting it at the End

Practitioners from some Yang-style schools pre-position the rear foot at the beginning of the movement, as illustrated in the transition from "Ward off Left" to "Ward off Right." First, these practitioners shift the weight from 70% on the left foot to 100% on the right foot. Next, they pivot the left foot 45° to the right. Then they shift 100% onto the pre-positioned left foot, turn to the right, and step with the right foot. Finally, the weight is shifted 70% to the right foot.

By contrast, Cheng Man-ch'ing taught his students to shift their weight 100% onto the left foot, step with the right foot, shift 70% into the right foot, and then pivot the left foot 45° to the right.

There are valid conceptual differences between the two ways of turning the foot: When the foot is pre-positioned, the turning part of the movement occurs *before* the shifting of the weight. Pivoting the foot at the end of the movement results in turning *after* shifting the weight. Practitioners of each method base their self-defense applications on a corresponding concept of the sequence in which shifting and turning occur.

When the foot is being preset, there is an extra back-and-forth shifting of the weight. While not seeming to conform to the principle of non-action, this extra shifting, nevertheless, substantially activates the flow of Ch'i.

By contrast, pivoting the foot at the end of the movement requires a much greater opening of the thigh joints while stepping. This latter method is much more difficult for beginners, but the opening (and closing) of the thigh joints improves flexibility and generates Ch'i in a different way.

I have practiced the pivoting method for more than twenty-four years and the pre-positioning method for more than ten years. I have found that each provides a substantial but different benefit. Both are certainly worthwhile.

T'AI CHI CH'UAN COMPARED TO "AEROBIC" EXERCISE

Today there is a strong emphasis on the importance of aerobic exercise. In aerobic exercise, stored energy is utilized through the chemical change of glycogen to water and carbon dioxide instead of intermediate waste products such as lactic acid. The term *aerobic* is used because it refers to a process wherein the utilization of oxygen is maximized. An analogy would be a stove in which gas is burned fully rather than partially. Examples of aerobic exercises are running, bicycling, fast walking, and swimming, when these are done for sufficiently long periods of time (one-half hour or more).

While aerobic exercise is highly beneficial, many of its most-sought-after cardiovascular benefits are also achieved by practicing T'ai Chi Ch'uan. There are two ways to exercise the cardiovascular system. One way is to place it under a stress for a period of time, thereby strengthening it. The other way is to relax the muscles and extraneous nerve impulses so that the cardiovascular system can be gently stimulated and be nourished by Ch'i.

Furthermore, when push-hands is practiced in a spirited manner with a challenging partner, it certainly can be regarded as an aerobic exercise and gives the best of both worlds.

OTHER TEACHINGS

Some practitioners of T'ai Chi Ch'uan are prone to extolling its virtues at the expense of other teachings. One should be open to all knowledge and not negatively characterize that which is not fully understood.

It has been my experience that being confronted with apparent contradictions of other disciplines and resolving them is the best way to learn. In the words of my teacher Harvey I. Sober, who has mastered a number of different academic disciplines and styles of martial arts and studied with many teachers, "Alternative ways are different—not necessarily wrong. To have studied only one interpretation is like having read only one book or heard only one piece of music."

Notes

1. Willi Apel, *Harvard Dictionary of Music,* The Belknap Press of Harvard University Press, Cambridge, MA, 1969.

2. See Robert H. Dreisbach, *Handbook of Poisoning,* Lange Medical Publications, Los Altos, CA, 1969, p. 155.

3. See, for example, Tseng Chiu-yien, *The Chart of Tai Chi Chuan,* Union Press Limited, 14, Dorset Crescent, Kowloon Tong, Kowloon, Hong Kong.

4. Robert W. Smith, *Chinese Boxing: Masters and Methods,* Kodansha International, Ltd., Tokyo, 1974, pp. 36–37.

5. Ibid., pp. 53–54.

CHAPTER 11

Push-Hands Basics

Invest in loss. Small loss: small dividend; large loss: large dividend.
—Cheng Man-ch'ing

After the beginning T'ai Chi Ch'uan student has completed the solo form and that form has been substantially corrected, the student is then taught push-hands. Push-hands involves reacting to the movements of another person according to a set of basic principles and is of such a level of difficulty that it is essential that the T'ai Chi principles of solo movement be first sufficiently assimilated.

In practicing push-hands, you become acutely aware of a partner's intentions and learn to control his balance as soon as he makes a movement. Controlling another's balance is accomplished by means of *neutralization.* Once your partner's movement is neutralized, you can *return* by pushing (the terms *neutralization* and *return* will be discussed later in this chapter under their respective headings). Substantial practice is necessary in order to achieve the strength, sensitivity, judgment, and timing required to neutralize and return effectively. Since, during practice, you must subdue your own ego, progress is slow and can be fraught with frustration, but the ultimate benefits are great.

There are two basic methods of push-hands practice: fixed-step push-hands and moving push-hands. Moving push-hands is more advanced.

In fixed-step push-hands, each partner's feet remain essentially glued to the same spot on the floor. Without this restriction, most beginners would evade their partner's attack by stepping away, thereby losing an opportunity to learn to neutralize.

Moving push-hands is an exercise that builds sensitivity to the opponent's intention to step forward, backward, or to the side.

One-Handed Push-Hands

You and your partner pair off in what is called a *harmonious 70-30* stance, which means that both of you assume a 70-30 stance with right feet forward or both with left feet forward (see chapter 7 for a discussion of stances). Your forward foot is a shoulder width apart from your partner's forward foot. The closeness of both partners to each other depends on the relative placement of their forward feet. This placement can vary to the extent indicated in Fig. 11-1. If each partner's right foot is forward, then the partners contact each other with their right wrists. (If their two left feet were forward, then their left wrists would make contact.) *A* attacks by extending his right hand toward *B*'s center. *B* defends by first shifting her weight back, without turning her body in either direction. After *A* has extended his arm toward *B*'s center, she then turns to the right, thereby deflecting his hand to her right. Thus, the defender deflects toward the side of her forward foot.

The reason that *B* initially moves straight back is that, if she deflected *A* to the right too early, he could fold his right arm and attack with his right

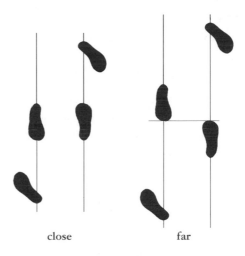

close   far

Fig. 11-1. *The range of relative placement of the partners' feet in push-hands. (Harmonious stance with right feet forward.)*

forearm. There are three reasons for deflecting toward the right (forward) leg: (1) It exposes the attacker's unprotected side (left arm useless) to the defender's strong side (left arm free). (2) The attacker is led into a position of imbalance (the double-weighted position). (3) The defender's center automatically moves back and to the left when she sits back on her left leg (her center of mass shifts toward her rear foot). Therefore, sitting back on her left foot will cause an attack to her center to miss and pass to her right. It can be seen that deflecting to the right is consistent with the sideways motion of your center away from the attack.

Next, *B* assumes the role of the attacker and shifts forward, extending her right hand toward *A*'s center. As *B* attacks, she turns back to the left so that her center is directed toward that of *A*. He responds in the same manner as she did, deflecting her hand to his right. During a complete cycle, the motion of the two hands, which never lose contact (*sticking*), is a counterclockwise oval, as viewed from above.

Note that it is important that your navel point directly toward your partner's center while you are pushing.

When your partner extends his forward hand to a substantial degree, his elbow presents a danger to you. Therefore, you must lightly contact his elbow with your other hand. Ways of contacting the opponent will be discussed later in this chapter.

Two-Handed Push-Hands

In two-handed push-hands, the movements "Ward Off," "Rollback," "Press," and "Push" (P'eng, Lu, Chi, and An), respectively, (collectively referred to as

"Grasping the Sparrow's Tail") are employed by each partner in a harmonious interplay of yielding and attacking movements. Cheng Man-ch'ing's second book[1] gives a good description of fixed-step, two-handed push-hands.

Moving Push-Hands

In moving push-hands, two people pair off as in stationary push-hands. Again, each person alternately attacks and then yields to the other's attack. But now, one partner may unexpectedly step forward with his rear foot. At the same time, the other partner steps backward with the corresponding foot to restore a harmonious stance. Or, one partner may initiate a step backward or to the side, in which case the other partner also steps correspondingly. You should practice moving push-hands only after you are able to deal with a strong push-hands attack *without* moving your feet.

BASIC CONCEPTS OF PUSH-HANDS

Concept of T'ai Chi

The concept of T'ai Chi (harmonious interplay of yin and yang) is the fundamental principle that underlies all push-hands movements; namely, when one partner attacks (yang), the other must neutralize (yin). A buildup of rigid muscular force is considered to be incorrect. Push-hands does not rely on brute strength but is based on "understanding force." If one partner does not yield but manifests rigidity, then the other partner can push but must neutralize first. The neutralization must not involve much force. The legendary maximum neutralizing force is "four ounces." This maximum, however, *does not* apply to the push, which can involve as much force as necessary.

Students find it very difficult to understand the special meanings of the terms *yield, neutralize,* and *softness* (correct force). Each time beginning students try to be soft, they immediately lose to more-advanced students. Seeing that their attempts to yield lead only to "defeat," beginners tend to lose faith in the efficacy of yielding. Additionally, beginning students find that pushing more-advanced students without rigid strength is of little use. Therefore, beginners tend to disbelieve that a push can succeed without involving contractive muscular force. Moreover, they always seem to be accused of being rigid when they feel they are not. All of these factors result in beginners reverting to the use of contractive muscular force and a consequent slowing of progress. Therefore, it is essential that beginning push-hands students be exposed to the concept of softness even though they may not yet be able to manifest it. They must suspend disbelief and, in the words of Cheng Man-ch'ing, "invest in loss." This approach will be elaborated upon later in this chapter, under *Attitude.*

Yielding

Yield means to permit the opponent to execute an attack and encounter only minimum resistance.

For a beginner, *yielding* tends to take the form of retreating further and further until 100% of the weight is on his rear leg. While beginners are thus easily pushed, this manner of retreating is still better than blocking or becoming rigid. Blocking or rigidly resisting an attack may work sometimes. However, the resistance will immediately alert a knowledgeable opponent, who will be able to circumvent and utilize it.

Yielding is said to occur when the part of the body that is attacked has a substantial component of motion in the same direction as the attack. It is permissible for the person who yields to allow a small force to be exerted by the attacker. However, it will be explained later that the smaller this force is, the greater will be the control over the opponent's balance. The beginner should think of yielding primarily as a means of attaining control over his own body. Certainly it is impossible to effectively control another's actions without first being able to control one's own actions. Of course, the beginner will get pushed a lot during this phase.

Neutralization

After students have become proficient at yielding, they should begin to work on neutralizing. The difference between yielding and neutralizing is subtle. Yielding merely involves moving with the opponent's attack to prevent force from building up. This movement does not necessarily place the opponent at a disadvantage or improve the position of the person who yields. Neutralizing, on the other hand, involves a yielding movement *plus a sideways deflection.* Here it is important to make the distinction between *deflection* and *blocking.* Deflection differs from blocking in that deflection interferes with the movement of the opponent as little as possible, whereas blocking is a clash in the attempt to punish or forcibly restrict the motion of the attacking limb. Blocking is not used in T'ai Chi Ch'uan.

Neutralization leads an attack away from one's center so that no harmful force can be exerted by the attacker. Neutralization also impairs the position of the attacker and momentarily breaks his balance and root. The attacker expects to meet resistance and braces himself to adjust his balance in terms of this expectation. When the expected resistance in the direction of the attack is absent, the attacker must momentarily readjust the forces to restore his balance. At that moment the attacker's position is weak, and he experiences confusion.

It can be seen that neutralizing requires a more refined level of processing and reacting than just yielding, which is merely passive. Neutralization requires a knowledge of the opponent's balance, an ability to sense where he is strong or weak, and the ability to lead him from strength to weakness.

One reason that neutralization is so difficult to master is that we tend to *sense our partner's strength and our own weakness* and focus only on those. To neutralize effectively, we must also sense and utilize the opposite, namely, *our own strength and our opponent's weakness.*

For a beginner, neutralizing involves a relatively large movement that makes him correspondingly weak. But, as neutralization is refined, it involves a movement so small that only an adept practitioner can observe it. In the highest stages of ability, the practitioner is able to continually neutralize and, thus, continually control the attacker's balance as soon as any movement is made by him. In fact, when his balance is initially broken, the attacker tends to lean on the person he is attacking to restore his balance. It is possible for an advanced practitioner to prevent the opponent from regaining his balance and to take advantage of even a tiny movement of the opponent to render him helpless.

Neutralization need not occur only during a defensive action but can also be part of an attack. If your attack is countered with resistance, you can neutralize this resistance to advantage. How a buildup of force was initiated is not as important as how that force is dealt with.

It may be of interest to relate something that happened to me shortly after I started learning push-hands. I was in the supermarket, and a woman accidentally bumped into me. As soon as I felt her contact me, I automatically neutralized the force, and, to our mutual surprise, she nearly fell to the floor. In thinking about it later, I realized what had happened. When she bumped into me, she expected a force to be exerted on her by me and depended on it for her balance. This force was absent because of the reflex response that I had developed from push-hands practice. Consequently, she lost her balance and started to lean on me to regain it. Had I continued to neutralize, she would have fallen. This experience gave me, as a beginner, an inkling of how neutralizing works.

Correct Force (Softness)

Softness is a concept about which there is a great deal of confusion and controversy. For some practitioners, push-hands practice involves the use of almost no force, whereas for others, practice involves tremendous force. How can we reconcile these apparently contradictory ways of practicing? The surprising fact is that *both ways of practicing are useful and complementary.* Consider the following explanation:

Some practitioners mistakenly believe that T'ai Chi Ch'uan does not involve strength. While it is true that the familiar contractive muscular strength that weight lifters develop should not be used, strength of a different type is cultivated and employed. This strength is developed by practicing sung. Sung involves a complete giving-in to gravity. In a state of sung, the muscles of the legs submit to being lengthened to their full extension without any attempt on their part to contract. Over a period of time, the leg muscles develop enormous springiness and strength. At the same time, the muscles of the upper body develop the ability to transmit a high degree of force by *extending*. The result is that when an opponent exerts force on such a practitioner, that force is immediately converted into potential energy of the stretched muscles of the practitioner's legs. At the optimal instant, this energy can be released through the upper body and back to the opponent with devastating effect. Correct force expands without obstruction or interruption upward from the soles of the feet, through the trunk of the body, and out through the extremities.

It can be seen that there are two aspects to correct force: (1) strength and (2) the subtle regulation of this strength. The strength aspect of T'ai Chi Ch'uan is developed through practicing the form in a state of sung and through practicing push-hands rooting with very powerful opponents. However, such practice alone is insufficient to achieve softness. The exclusive use of a large amount of force deprives practitioners of opportunities to learn sensitivity and timing. Similarly, those who practice never letting force build up develop sensitivity and timing but are not able to deal with an opponent who roots and uses muscular force, let alone correct force.

Thus, ideal practice must eventually cultivate the entire range of force, so that the practitioner develops not only sensitivity, timing, and the ability to neutralize with minimum force but also the ability to receive and return the energy of a strong opponent.

Rooting and Redirecting

Rooting and redirecting is a manner of dealing with an incoming push by sinking your weight into your feet (sung), becoming immovable (rooting), and subtly pushing back in another direction (redirecting). The redirecting is done in such a manner that the person who is pushing finds that he loses his balance if he continues. The mechanics of rooting and redirecting are explained in terms of Newton's third law as follows (see chapter 3 for a full discussion of Newton's third law): When A attempts to push B, he does so by exerting a force on her. B can choose to neutralize that force by means of a yielding action. Or, she can choose to allow that force to build up and simultaneously exert a judiciously placed and directed small counter force on A. In the latter case, there are now two separate forces on A. One force is the reaction to his initial force, and the other is the counter force exerted by B. The net effect of these two forces is, by design, in A's direction of weakness. Now if A continues his attack, he will lose his balance. In response, A will involuntarily retract his original force. Thus, A's attack is neutralized. Of course, for this manner of neutralizing to work, it is necessary to know just the right counter force to exert.

Rooting and redirecting has a valid place in push-hands practice. By rooting and dealing with a strong partner, you learn to use the right kind of force in both receiving and returning. You also learn where the opponent is weak, because there is no reservation about using a relatively large amount of force to test the opponent's suspected weakness. With practice, you will eventually develop (a) a keen awareness of the strength or weakness of your own position and that of the opponent and (b) the ability to control the opponent's balance with very small amounts of force.

Professor Cheng discouraged his beginning students from using rooting and redirecting techniques during push-hands practice. He wanted us to develop the ability to neutralize by means of yielding, which he considered to be of primary importance. I think that he did not want to see his students "Sumo wrestling" with each other. He preferred that we develop subtle and higher-level skills that we would not be likely to otherwise learn. While Cheng discouraged rooting and redirecting, he strongly emphasized rooting while practicing the T'ai Chi Ch'uan form. Thus, students who followed Cheng's instruction would have achieved a good level of sung by the time they were ready to learn push-hands rooting. Unfortunately, Cheng died in 1975, before the majority of his students in New York City were ready to be taught much else beyond rudimentary neutralization. Consequently, many of his students consider rooting and redirecting a wrong avenue and continue to avoid it.

Nevertheless, Cheng would occasionally demonstrate rooting. On page 32 of *T'ai Chi Ch'uan, Body and Mind,* published by the T'ai Chi Ch'uan Association to commemorate its third anniversary in 1968, there is a photograph of Cheng resisting the push of four men, one of whom was the late Patrick Watson, a very large and strong person.

During routine push-hands play with his more advanced students, Cheng would, at times, meet their soft push with a springy firmness that would stop the student in his tracks. Next, Cheng would subtly absorb and expand in quick succession, sending the student flying with enormous speed. Cheng's movements would be so internal that they would be barely visible.

On the numerous occasions that I did push-hands with William C. C. Chen, he never once presented any resistance. He is so quick and flexible that he was given the nickname "wasp waist" when he was in China. This nickname is aptly deserved. He is so elusive that one time he seemed to disappear entirely, only to reappear behind me and give me a totally unexpected push.

Harvey I. Sober manifests rooting and redirecting on a high level and encourages his students to learn these skills as *well* as neutralization by yielding. Sober's ability to disturb an opponent's balance is so highly refined that he can do so with the slightest force. When he merely touches me while I am doing my best to uproot him, I feel all of my energy being drained away. My *physics* explanation is that his light touch is so precisely directed and threatening to my balance that I sense that my continuing with the slightest attacking movement will result in a complete loss of my balance. Thus, I experience his action as a draining of my energy. Since such an ability seems to require more than just a physical aspect, what is involved may be beyond the ability of physics to explain.

Returning

After students have learned to neutralize, they then work on returning. Returning means that when the attacker is off balance, you exert a force on him in just the right direction, in just the right amount, and at just the right instant. In the case of push-hands practice, if this force is properly applied, it results in an *uproot.* An uproot occurs when the opponent involuntarily springs into the air with both feet off the ground. If only one foot moves, it is a partial uproot.

In the case of actual combat, the force of the return is very large (a strike) and can simultaneously uproot and severely injure the opponent. It is effective because the blow is centered and delivered at the instant that maximizes a transfer of force.

Note that it is absolutely necessary to neutralize before pushing. Pushing without first neutralizing requires brute strength, whereas a correct push involves a clean, spring-like action.

Receiving Energy

According to Cheng Man-ch'ing, the highest level that a T'ai Chi Ch'uan devotee can attain is the ability to receive energy.[2] To paraphrase Cheng's explanation, *receiving energy* is different from deflecting a force to the side, which only works for small or moderate forces. When a highly trained opponent attacks with full force, it is very difficult, if not impossible, to neutralize the attack by deflecting it. Instead, the defender receives the energy of the attacker by attracting it to his body, like iron to a magnet. The defender's body must internally act like a spring that compresses until the total energy of the opponent is stored. This energy can then be returned to the opponent with impressive results.

In order for you to receive energy, it is necessary that your body be capable of being totally empty (sung) and so strong so that it can withstand the consequent intake of the opponent's energy. The state of emptiness is achieved by practicing the solo form assiduously over many years, with a mind toward achieving the greatest degree of inner liquefaction and connectedness. The strength is achieved by practicing push-hands rooting regularly for years with challenging partners. While it is important to practice evasive action by deflecting with less than four ounces, such practice, alone, will not develop the strength required for receiving energy.

PUSH-HANDS PRINCIPLES

Use of Minimum Force when Neutralizing

The use of minimum force when neutralizing is essential in controlling the opponent's balance. However, it is also important from the point of view of sensitivity. *Weber's law* (see chapter 3) states that the minimum perceptible increase in a stimulus is proportional to the intensity of that stimulus. Thus, if you contact the opponent with a heavy touch, a given change in contact force will be much less noticeable to you than with a lighter touch. The lighter the touch, the greater the sensitivity. In addition, the lighter the touch, the less it will alert the opponent.

Unfortunately, many students of push-hands tend to be competitive and *habitually* use an excessive force to thwart an incoming attack. When two practitioners *A* and *B* pair off to do push-hands and *A* resists, *B* will do either one of two things: (1) *B* will use more force, in which case the use of force in attacking and in defending continually escalates. Or, (2) *B* will suspend her initial attack rather than use force. Then *A* feels successful in thwarting *B*'s attack and becomes more likely to resist future attacks.

It is the job of the teacher to monitor students' use of force and intervene when brute force is employed in the name of neutralization. The teacher must inculcate cooperation and, consequently, a balance in the use of strength and lightness.

Sticking

Sticking has many facets. In simplest terms, *sticking* means to maintain physical and mental contact with the opponent. For example, when the opponent's hand comes within your range, a correct response is to make contact with his wrist. In fact, the more points of contact, the better. When there are multiple contact points, it is easier to control the magnitude, direction, and line of action of the force exerted on the opponent. This control is essential for optimal neutralizing and returning. The wrist, hand, forearm, elbow, and shoulder are effective parts of the body to use for contact. At times any part of the body can be effectively used to trap a vulnerable part of the opponent. However, allowing the opponent to aggressively make contact with the trunk of your body is usually to be avoided because the trunk is more vulnerable and more difficult to maneuver than the hands, wrists, arms, elbows, and shoulders. Moreover, in a fighting situation, once a skilled opponent is touching your body, he can use an internal motion to deliver a penetrating blow without removing his hand. This release of internal energy is termed *Fa Chin.*

An important reason for maintaining light contact is that it provides a sensitive indication of any change in the opponent's balance and intention. In a self-defense situation, it is more difficult for the opponent to strike you with a limb that is continually in contact with your arm or hand, which can follow its motion and deflect it.

"Listening"

One of the most important aspects of push-hands is to develop sensitivity to your partner's intentions, balance, and movement. This sensitivity is developed through *listening.* Listening has nothing to do with physical hearing through the ears but refers to an analogous attentiveness and processing with all of the senses— possibly including extra-sensory perception. Even before there is physical contact with the opponent, the advanced practitioner knows more about the opponent than the opponent knows about himself. The following story about an Aikido master will illustrate the degree of attunement to the intentions of others that is possible.

In the early 1970's I attended a demonstration given by a tenth-degree Aikido master. The demonstration took place in the rectangular courtyard of a church. The audience was seated on all four sides of the courtyard. The master stood in the center and spoke in his native Japanese, which was then translated into English. At that time, I had little knowledge of martial arts or martial arts customs, and I did not realize that this master's seemingly immodest remarks were really a conservative prelude to amazing feats of ability that would follow. I ignorantly said to myself, "If he doesn't stop bragging about his abilities, I am going to leave." As if in response to my thoughts, he slowly and deliberately turned 180 degrees to face my direction and, without looking at me directly, said, "Never look directly into the eyes of a person who confronts you—you will create an enemy." Next he said, "I want you all to know that I am *totally protected*. If anyone so much as has a bad thought about me, I know it immediately." Astounded, I was now glued to his every word and action.

As the demonstration progressed, this master reached a point where he was throwing multiple attackers (who were third- to fifth-degree black belts) to the mat without even touching them. He had become so attuned to their movement, and they became so afraid of being overcome by him, that, as soon as they made the slightest movement, he threw them with only the *threat* of a technique.

Non-Action

In any situation, a particular course of action should be initiated only if doing so can be expected to produce a clear-cut advantage. Otherwise, it is better to do nothing. Alternatively stated, "don't overdo." In push-hands, this principle of non-action applies both to quantity of force and quantity of motion.

With regard to force, any excess corresponds to unnecessary commitment and reduces sensitivity (Weber's law). With regard to motion, any excess is an unnecessary commitment and reduces the element of surprise. The goal then is to deflect to the minimum degree (principle of non-action).

The manner in which the principle of non-action is applied in practice is as follows: when my partner attacks, he does so by exerting a force. I must move in such a manner that this force never becomes larger than a few ounces. As he tries to exert this force, he is led into a position of weakness, and I, in turn, acquire a position of strength. This can be outwardly accomplished in two stages of expertise.

1. During the earlier stages of training, students should strive to release tension to the degree that the most gentle touch of the partner sets their own body into a yielding motion. That is, the partner's force physically causes the yielding action. This *passive* type of response must first be developed because beginners have a strong tendency to initiate a defensive action either without regard to the partner's action or as a result of an incorrectly anticipated action. Beginning push-hands students first react by bracing against any incoming attack. Once they learn that resisting is incorrect, they next attempt to yield by impulsively pulling or pushing various parts of their body. Acting on a preconceived idea of what the opponent will do *before he does it,* the beginner becomes fixated on a response even though that response may become inappropriate after

a change in the opponent's movements occurs. During practice, you should not pull and push various parts of your body using muscular actions. Instead, arrange an inner condition of relaxation and total connectedness. Then, your body will be moved by the force that the opponent exerts—no matter how slight that force is. The classics say that the whole body must be so perfectly balanced that an insect alighting on it will set it into motion. This statement implies that the minute force of the insect's feet is the propelling agent.

2. During more advanced stages, you will know the intention of your partner before he acts, and you will *actively* respond by *leading* him into weakness. When the opponent starts to exert force on you, you must sense his intention, direction, strength, and weakness as well as your own strength and weakness. Of the spectrum of possible movements, you must know that which will maximize both your strength and your opponent's weakness. Your movement *is* actually initiated by the opponent rather than yourself; if it precedes the actions of the opponent, it does so only as a result of a highly developed ability to listen and react. Such preemptive movement does not violate the principle of non-action. In the T'ai Chi Classics, Wu Yu-Hsiang says, "If others (opponents) don't move, I don't move. If others move slightly, I move first."[3] This seemingly paradoxical statement is meaningful in terms of the above explanation.

Replacement

Whenever there is contact between one part of your body and a part of the opponent's body, it is possible to make a subtle substitution. For example, imagine that you and your partner *P* pair off in a harmonious stance, each with the right foot forward and right hand forward and with right wrists touching. You can replace your right wrist with your left wrist as follows: First raise your left wrist to touch *P*'s right wrist. Now both of your wrists contact *P*'s right wrist. As you release the pressure of your right wrist, correspondingly increase the pressure of your left wrist. Once the pressure exerted by your right wrist decreases to zero, you can remove that wrist entirely. While *P*'s visual impression will be that a change has occurred, it will be difficult for him to react to this change because the tactile sensation will have been constant.

Folding

One valuable principle is that of folding. There are instances when certain parts of your body contact corresponding parts of the opponent's body, and those contact points are not optimal for the exertion of an uprooting force. An undesirable option would be to break contact and make new contact at better locations. However, breaking contact is dangerous because (a) its discontinuity acts as a signal to the opponent that something is about to occur, and (b) it creates an opportunity for the opponent to react freely. Instead of breaking contact, it is better to maintain contact and fold in such a manner that new contact points are established. Then, the original contact can be safely withdrawn. For example, assume that you are contacting the opponent with both of your hands on the opponent's chest, and he turns to his left, bringing his right hand in contact with your left wrist in an attempt to dislodge it from his body. One response is to *permit* him to move your wrist by simultaneously turning to your right and bringing your left forearm in contact with his right upper arm. Now, you can push him with your left forearm.

Opposite Palms

The principle of opposite palms governs the ideal way to exert force for a given stance. For example, if the weight is 100% on your right leg, then using your right hand to push the opponent will cause you to be weak and unbalanced. This weakness occurs because the right side of your body must be more or less motionless if balance is to be maintained, but the strongest action requires the most bodily movement. Therefore, the weighted side of your body is the weaker side to use for pushing or striking. In conventional boxing, fighters use the fist on the weighted side for the jab, which is not powerful but annoying and fast. Once the opponent is off balance or dazed, then the fist *opposite* the weighted leg is employed for the "knockout."

Contacting an Opponent

It is important that correct contact be made. The usual points of contact are the wrists, palms, and elbows. The combinations are as follows:

1. The back of A's wrist contacts the back of B's wrist. This is the manner in which partners contact each other in one-handed push-hands or in the "Press" position in two-handed push-hands. The best point of contact is not the back of B's hand but the end of the bone of her arm. When A contacts the back of B's hand, there is the danger that B will suddenly bend her wrist and slip off. Moreover, when A uses the back of his hand for contact, tension is needed to keep his wrist from bending, whereas using the end of his arm bone allows his hand to relax. Therefore both partners should strive for mutual contact of the bones.

2. The hollow of the palm of A's hand contacts B's elbow. This is the manner in which partners contact each other in two-handed push-hands with A in the "Push" position and B in the "Rollback" position. Here the palm and elbow "mate" in a manner similar to that of a ball-and-socket joint. This contact produces the greatest control of the elbow.

   If the contact of A's hand is made below B's elbow, B's elbow can escape by "walking" over A's wrist.

   If the contact of A's hand is made above B's elbow, her elbow can escape by slipping under his wrist.

3. The hollow of the palm of A's hand contacts the back of B's wrist. This is the manner in which partners contact each other in two-handed push-hands with A in the "Push" position and B in the "Rollback" position. Here the palm and wrist "mate" as a ball and socket.

If the contact of *A*'s hand is made above *B*'s wrist, her wrist can escape by levering over his wrist.

4. *A*'s elbow contacts *B*'s elbow. Again, this is the manner in which partners contact each other in two-handed push-hands with *A* in the "Rollback" position and *B* in the "Push" position.

It is a good idea to work on perfecting these basic principles of contact for a period at the beginning of each two-handed push-hands practice session.

Neutralizing Before Returning

The beginning push-hands student tends to execute a shove as soon as he senses his partner's center or imbalance. Those who do not cultivate sensing and controlling another's balance during each moment of the push develop an ability to push only by using speed and brute force. In order to reach the highest level, however, you must be able to cause the opponent to become off balance and then use this imbalance to uproot him.

MISCELLANEOUS CONCEPTS

Importance of Stance

Assume that the practitioner is in a 70-30 stance with the left foot forward. Consider a line L' drawn from the weight center C_F of the forward foot to the weight center C_R of the rear foot (see Fig. 11-2). (Note that L'' is not the length L of the stance.) Because the weight is 70% on the forward foot, the center of gravity is located at point p on L', 70% of the distance from C_R to C_F. When the weight is shifted 100% onto the rear leg, the center of gravity shifts along line L' until it is directly over C_R. There is a sideways component of motion of the body to the right a distance of 70% of the width of the 70-30 stance or, equivalently, 70% of a shoulder width. Thus, by sitting back from a 70-30 position to a 100% position, you automatically shift toward the side of your rear leg, even if no other action occurs. Therefore, the width of the stance determines the extent of the sideways motion and is critical for neutralization. (Other benefits of the proper-width 70-30 stance that have already been mentioned are stability and the ability to turn.) Similarly, there is a corresponding rearward motion of the body equal to 70% of the length of the stance when your weight is shifted back from a 70-30 position to a 100%

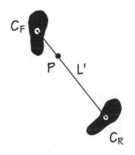

Fig. 11-2. *Variation of the center of mass in the 70-30 stance. As the weight is shifted from the 70-30 stance to the 100% stance, the enter of mass shifts from point P to C_R.*

position. Thus, the longer the stance, the longer the rearward movement during neutralization. Since the lower the stance, the longer it becomes, practitioners constantly work on sinking into lower and lower stances.

Circles

Why are the deflections of T'ai Chi Ch'uan circular? The answer partly involves the concept of continuity. When A attacks and B deflects perpendicularly, according to the T'ai Chi Ch'uan principles, there must be no discontinuity in the force exerted. Discontinuity implies impulsiveness and gaps in attentiveness and telegraphs one's intentions to the opponent. A circular deflection builds up the deflecting force gradually rather than impulsively (as in hard styles). Towards the end of the deflection B is exerting the maximum force (albeit small). Exerting the maximum force at the end is best from the point of view of leverage because the more A extends, the more effective is B's sideways push. Also, if B waits until the last moment, it is less likely that A will realize what is happening and be able to adjust.

Therefore, the initial path of A's attack is straight, and its direction is gradually changed in a circular manner.

Equilibrium

There are three types of equilibrium—stable, unstable, and neutral. To distinguish these types of equilibrium, imagine a cone, similar to an ice-cream cone (without the ice cream). Stable equilibrium is illustrated by the cone placed on its circular base. When an object is in stable equilibrium, any displacement will cause its center of mass to rise. Therefore when the cone is displaced and then released, it will return to its initial position.

Unstable equilibrium is illustrated by the cone balanced on its point. When an object is in unstable equilibrium, any displacement will cause its center of mass to be lowered. Therefore when the cone is displaced and then released, it will fall.

Neutral equilibrium is illustrated by the cone placed on its side. When an object is in neutral equilibrium, any displacement will cause its center of mass to be neither raised nor lowered. Therefore when the cone is displaced and then released, it will roll but not fall. (See the section on balance in chapter 3 for a fuller discussion of equilibrium.)

Your equilibrium should be stable when still and neutral when in motion. Moreover, one should always try to make the opponent's equilibrium unstable and cause him to move in the direction of increasing instability.[4]

Equilibrium is approximately unstable when the weight is 100% on one foot. It becomes even less stable when the weight is 100% on one foot but is concentrated on one part of the foot (e.g., the ball or heel). There is also a component of instability in the direction perpendicular to the line joining the weight centers of the two feet. This is the double-weighted direction (see chapter 3).

It is possible to transform the unidirectional instability of a double-weighted opponent into an omnidirectional instability as follows: Push into your partner's double-weighted direction. As he loses balance, he will naturally reposition one foot. During the instant that he lifts that foot, his equilibrium becomes increasingly unstable in all directions, and he can be easily pushed into his original direction of stability.

Action and Reaction

Newton's third law states that if body A exerts a force (the *action*) on body B, then B exerts an equal but opposite force (the *reaction*) on A. One consequence of this law is that it is impossible for an attacker to exert a force on you without your exerting the same force on the attacker.

The idea in push-hands is to control the attacker's force by adjusting the force you exert on the attacker. The Chinese classics say that a force of 1,000 pounds can be deflected by four ounces.

In push-hands, it frequently arises that one student accuses his or her partner of being "heavy." The answer is that it takes *two* to be heavy. One person cannot be held solely responsible for the use of too much force. However, the attacker can be held *more* responsible in the following sense: The person defending must follow, which is more difficult. On the other hand, if the person defending is *actively* using force rather than merely *unable* to neutralize, *he* is more responsible. It is important to be able to analyze the situation rather than blame your partner (or, for that matter, yourself).

Newton's Third Law and the Push-Hands Uproot

When the opponent is properly uprooted, both of his feet leave the ground, as if lifted by a puff of air. While it is not hard to understand how an opponent can occasionally be uprooted through the use of a large amount of force, the question naturally arises of how it is possible for a small person to lift someone who weighs 150 pounds or more completely into the air *without* a comparably large force. Using a force less than the weight of the lifted person seems to violate the laws of physics. Here is an explanation based on Newton's third law:

When A attempts to push B with a force of 10 pounds, A intuitively expects that she will, by Newton's third law, push back on him with a reaction force of 10 pounds. If this reaction were the only horizontal force on him, he would no longer be in equilibrium. Therefore, he pushes back on the floor with his foot with a frictional force of 10 pounds to maintain balance. The reaction to the 10-pound frictional force of A on the floor is a 10-pound frictional force of the floor on A in the forward direction. Now he can push on her and still remain in equilibrium. But, let us assume that she neutralizes his push. This means that he does not get a chance to exert a 10-pound force on her. However, he expected the force to be exerted and has arranged things so that the floor exerts a forward 10-pound frictional force on himself. Thus, there is an unbalanced forward force on him. Feeling that the floor is now pushing him forward, he adjusts involuntarily by using his forward foot to exert (a) a downward force on the floor and (b) a frictional force on the floor in the forward direction. The reaction to the downward force is the upward force of the floor on his forward foot. This adjustment keeps him from rotating forward. The reaction to the forward frictional force on the floor is the frictional force of the floor on him in his rearward direction. This reaction keeps him from accelerating forward.

If *B* now exerts a (small) rearward force on *A* just as he is reacting to his momentary imbalance, he will go flying backward. At the same time he will also be rotating backward. If *A* did nothing more, he would land with his back on the floor. Sensing this danger, he must react immediately.

The only thing that *A* can now do to avoid rotating backward is push the floor forcibly downward with his rear foot before his center of gravity extends behind it. The closer his center of gravity is to his rear foot, the more force he must use. The reaction to the force exerted by his rear foot on the floor is an upward force of the floor on him. All of *A*'s actions are involuntary. Now he is no longer rotating backward but is air-borne. This is the push-hands *uproot* described in terms of physics.

As just mentioned, the uproot is most effective when the center of gravity of the person being pushed is close to his rear leg. Thus, it is best to neutralize an opponent's push early on, so that he will lose balance before his center of mass is far forward of the rear leg. Similarly, it is not wise to start the push until the attacker has shifted to the rear. If the push is initiated too early, an uproot will be difficult.

In order to master the art of uprooting the opponent, much time must be spent in sensing all aspects of the process. The sequence is so subtle and short-lived that no amount of practice without an understanding of what is involved can be expected to result in mastery. One problem is that it is a tremendous temptation for the student to use muscular force to get a result instead of "investing in loss" over a long period of time. It is very important that students cooperate with one another so that both partners can reinforce the correct principles.

Controlling the Opponent's Balance

When there is physical contact between you and an opponent, it is possible to make him lose his balance even if he does not make an aggressive move. (In fact, on the higher levels of T'ai Chi Ch'uan it is possible to control another's balance even before physical contact is made.) Control of the opponent's balance is accomplished by minutely regulating and changing the force exerted during contact in such a manner that he becomes momentarily but involuntarily dependent upon you for his balance.

Let us see how this control is accomplished. When you apply a light pressure, the opponent must momentarily adjust his balance. One way that he can adjust is by bracing his feet against the floor. However, if you are aware of the opponent's imbalance, *you* can supply the needed adjustment by allowing him to brace against you. This adjustment places him in a state of balance that *you* control. Then, when you release the contact pressure, he will again lose his balance.

If the pressure is suddenly decreased to zero, he will quickly realize that he cannot depend on you for support and balance. Thus, a sudden decrease is to be avoided. Rather, if you release the force noticeably at first and then at a decreasing rate, the opponent will continually be encouraged to expect that he can regain his balance by leaning just a bit more on you. In this case he will be led increasingly into a state wherein you control his balance. This is the desired effect. In fact, if properly executed, this neutralization will cause him to become stuck to you, as if by glue, and consequently be under your control.

Note that it does not matter whether the original contact or movement is initiated by you or by the opponent.

More than one neutralization can occur at the same time. Often, when an opponent contacts you, there are two or three points of contact, each of which must be neutralized in order to control his balance. Success depends upon your ability to control the pressure on him.

This control was a skill that Cheng Man-ch'ing had mastered. When I touched him or he touched me, I had an immediate and continuing feeling of helplessness. It seemed as though he could prolong my helplessness indefinitely. When he was ready, he would send me flying as though I were lifted by a puff of air. The only contact that I felt was a warm, soft hand. There was never any noticeable force, and there was always a feeling that his control of me was absolutely precise. There was also a feeling on my part of extreme fear of becoming airborne that way. Whenever anyone tried to push Cheng, he was able to continuously neutralize by very slight movements. He would neutralize in such a manner that he never really moved backward—or, if he did move one part backward, another part would advance to compensate.

There is a legend about certain T'ai Chi Ch'uan masters who were able to catch birds with their bare hands. Once caught, a bird would be allowed to perch on the master's finger but be unable to fly away. The explanation is as follows: A bird cannot lift its wings without simultaneously exerting an additional downward force on its perch with its feet. The masters were sensitive enough to sense and neutralize this force, thereby preventing the bird from raising its wings. If you have a chance to see a crow or other large bird walking on the ground, watch how it crouches and presses downward when it prepares to spread its wings to take flight.

T'i Fang

The T'ai Chi Ch'uan uproot involves a technique of energy release termed *t'i fang*. T'i fang employs a subtle neutralization in addition to the main neutralization just described. T'i fang involves eliciting a minute resistance on the part of the attacker and then neutralizing that resistance. Once the attacker feels himself falling forward, in addition to pressing the ground with the toes of his forward foot, he will attempt to lean on you to regain his balance. Ideally, you will allow him to exert a small force on you, and, just before he regains his balance, you will let up slightly, causing him to lose his balance again. This time, however, it is different because now you are in control of his balance and have mobilized intrinsic energy for a push.

The t'i fang accomplishes a number of purposes:

1. It causes the attacker to involuntarily exert a slight force on you during the push, making it harder for him to neutralize.

2. It provides a subtle test that fine-tunes the magnitude, timing, and direction of your push.

3. It increases the attacker's confusion by nullifying his repeated attempts to regain balance. He will tend to repeat the same gross movement to regain balance as he did the first time even though his balance is not as far off as he experiences it to be or as it was just after the first neutralization. This sets him up for a much more effective push.

4. Since you are in control of the attacker, the direction of the push need not be opposite to the original direction of attack.

5. It gives you a chance to practice sensing the attacker's balance under controlled conditions.

I note here that Cheng Man-ch'ing told us that there should be *three* pushes. I take his words to mean that there is one main neutralization of the opponent's initial attack and two subsequent minor neutralizations for fine tuning.

The t'i fang is a method of controlling the opponent's balance and of fine tuning that control so that, on the final push, the opponent is exactly in unstable equilibrium (minimum force).

Eventually, the neutralization occurs over a very short amount of time—only that required for the attacker to experience his own imbalance. When the neutralization occurs, the attacker adjusts by exerting a force on the floor with his forward foot to keep from falling forward. The defender responds almost immediately, so that the attacker hardly gets off balance. However, the attacker's reaction on the floor is based on an expectation of needing to exert the full force required to keep himself from falling. Because everything happens so fast, the attacker cannot release the force he is exerting with his forward foot fast enough. Thus he over-reacts with an excessive force to an extremely short-lived imbalance. This causes him to be uprooted. The job of the T'ai Chi Ch'uan practitioner is to become so highly attuned to the opponent's imbalance and his reaction to that imbalance, that the practitioner can take full advantage of it by pushing at exactly the best time and in the best direction. Practice over a long period of time, with conscious understanding of the underlying principles, is of paramount importance.

Examples of T'i Fang

Example 1. Consider the following situation: *A* and *B* are in a harmonious 70-30 stance with their right feet forward. *B*'s left hand is contacting *A*'s upper right arm. *B*'s right hand is contacting *A*'s left wrist, which is against *A*'s chest. *B* would like to push *A* with her left hand because this push would be more powerful (principle of opposite palms). However if *B* were to push with her left hand now, *A* could easily root into his rear leg or, preferably, sit back and neutralize. Alternatively, if *B* were to push with her right hand into *A*'s double-weighted position, she would lack power. More importantly, that push would at most cause *A* to reposition one foot—hardly an uproot! To push properly, *B* must first apply a modest pressure on *A*'s chest with her right hand in his double-weighted direction. When *B* lets up, *A* will momentarily lose his balance. Then, while *A* is adjusting to this imbalance, *B* can successfully push with her left hand in a powerful manner. This t'i fang induces the opponent to exert a pressure on you, which you then neutralize.

Example 2. Assume that *A* and *B* are again in a harmonious 70-30 stance with their right feet forward. *A* attacks *B*'s neck with his right hand. *B* contacts *A*'s right wrist with her right hand and sits back, pulling his right hand into his double-weighted direction. Then she uses her left hand, contacting the right side of his chest, to push him in the direction opposite to his original attack.

Note that a pull and a push are mutually equivalent in terms of the effect of unbalancing the opponent.

Mobilizing Intrinsic Energy

For you to neutralize the opponent's attack and return swiftly and unexpectedly, it is necessary to slightly advance your body toward him while simultaneously neutralizing with the parts of your body that are touching him. This type of action is illustrated by the motion of the arms relative to the body in the "Push" movement in the form. Here, your body initially retreats while your hands do not, and then your body moves forward while your hands "float." Toward the end of the movement, your hands and arms become connected to your body, so that energy can be released.

Stepping In

There are three methods of stepping in:

1. When the weight is shifted onto the forward foot, the rear foot takes a small step forward, thereby creating a shortened stance. Then when the weight is shifted onto the rear foot the forward foot can take a small step forward. The stepping of the forward foot is coincident with the neutralization prior to a push.

   It is possible to take two or more of these small steps in succession.

2. When the weight is shifted onto the rear foot, the forward foot takes a small step forward. This step is coincident with the neutralization prior to a push.

   Again, it is possible to take two or more steps in succession.

3. When the weight is on the forward foot, that foot is then lifted and takes a (committed) step forward. The rear foot then slides forward to adjust the length of the stance. At the moment that the forward foot is off the floor, the body is "falling" forward. Therefore, this method of stepping is dangerous and should not be routinely used.

Grabbing

Grabbing is considered an unwise action in the practice of push-hands or self-defense for a variety of reasons. Grabbing involves a forceful contact by clenching the fingers. Therefore, the person being grabbed is very likely to become aware of the grabber's intentions and escape through the "gate" (the opening between the thumb and forefinger). This escape can result in a lot of momentum being imparted to the escaping limb, which, if properly circled, can result in a very dangerous strike to the grabber. While strikes are not permitted in push-hands, practicing an action that leaves you open to a strike is a poor idea.

Aside from the fact that grabbing is not subtle and telegraphs the grabber's intentions, grabbing involves a mental fixation and intention that is difficult to release or modify. That is, grabbing is a strong commitment and is not "being in the moment." It is usually easy to use the committed hand of the person who grabs to lead him into the direction of his greatest weakness.

Instead of grabbing, it is better to develop the ability to entrap the arms, elbows, and wrists of the opponent without clenching the fingers. This entrapment is accomplished by means of gentle pressure at strategic places—with any combination of hands, wrists, and body exerting pressure, all operating in concert. In this manner, you can subtly control your opponent without unnecessarily committing yourself or alerting him.

Note that there is a big difference between a grab and the locks of Ch'in Na. Grabbing involves the use of muscular strength and a fixation of intent. Locking involves following the opponent's movement and knowing how to take advantage of his weakness using leverage and superior position.

Pulling

Pulling is different from grabbing because it does not involve fixation, muscular strength, or undue commitment. Pulling involves a momentary grip using the thumb and, at most, *one* finger. The only time it is appropriate to pull an opponent is when he is off balance or overextended. Otherwise the opponent can defend by moving with the pull, stepping in, and pushing the person who pulls. Pulling an opponent towards yourself is very dangerous. Only pull toward the side and, then, toward the person's double-weighted direction.

Use of Speed

During push-hands, some practitioners routinely wait for an opening or imbalance and ferociously attack with great speed. Such a manner of attacking frequently results in an uproot because it is difficult for the partner to react so quickly.

Unfortunately, attacking with speed during push-hands practice results in a lost opportunity for both partners. Neither partner can possibly follow the sequence of events mentally. If, instead, things are done slowly, so that the person being attacked is allowed to process the events and react more correctly, then each partner will be more able to adjust to every change. The situation can then be used for learning rather than competition. A properly executed push involves controlling the balance of the opponent and can be done slowly. It should not depend on taking your partner by surprise by use of speed.

Of course, it is occasionally good to be subjected to speedy attacks in order to learn your limits.

Push-Hands Versus Self-Defense

While push-hands is not self-defense per se, it provides an important foundation and conditioning that, when supplemented by self-defense training, leads one to a high level of ability. The ability to neutralize and return, to read the intentions of the opponent, and to move with power and precision but with minimum action are of great value.

Aside from the obvious absence of striking, kicking, sweeping, and grabbing, push-hands has a set of ground rules that must be followed if progress is to be made. As has been previously emphasized, one of the most important facets of push-hands is to be able to control the opponent's balance without the use of rigid muscular force.

While both partners may not expect to be punched, kicked, or struck, basic principles of fighting must be adhered to. For example, it is important to interpose a wrist, forearm, or elbow between an attacking limb of the opponent and your body or face at all times. This adherence promotes an awareness of vulnerability that would be present in a fighting situation. It is the obligation of each partner to point out by appropriate means (such as feigning) when the other repeatedly leaves himself open in an obvious manner.

Occasionally, push-hands turns into the kind of sparring found in other martial arts. It is essential that this changeover occur by mutual consent.

When I was a student at William C. C. Chen's school, I was doing push-hands with another student whom I had never seen before. He probably had studied Judo because, at one point, he unexpectedly stepped behind me, placed his arm across my neck, and tried to trip me using his hip. At that time I had never experienced this type of move before. Nevertheless, I reacted by emptying the side in contact with his hip, stepping in, and pushing him against the wall. He hit the wall with a very loud sound caused by the loose paneling lining the walls. The sound prompted everyone in the room to stop to see what had happened. I was just as surprised as everyone else. Thinking about this encounter later, I realized that, though I never practiced neutralizing with the lower part of my body, I had automatically transferred this ability.

Just as some sparring techniques have a limited appropriateness in push-hands, pushing can be used to a limited degree in sparring. When I was in a sparring class at Chen's school, I wanted to apply what I knew about pushing. I had been trained by Professor Cheng never to push anyone if there was no wall to stop that person from flying dangerously into the room. Because of my cautiousness and the nature of sparring, it was a long time before I found a valid opportunity to give my partner a good push. When I finally took advantage of an opportunity, again, the sound of my partner hitting the wall paneling caused everyone to stop and look. My partner was embarrassed and later complained to Chen about my pushing him. At this point, Chen called the class together and quietly explained to everyone that pushing was an appropriate technique to use while sparring.

"Taking Punches"

The logical extension of rooting is the ability to receive, without harm, the full force of an opponent's punch in a fighting (not a push-hands) situation. Chen termed this ability *taking punches*. Chen would encourage his students to hit him with full force on just about any part of his body. He wanted to provide a real target for his students to hit, and, by feeling the impact, he would know how to correct the student's punch to increase it's power. As his student, I hit him numerous times (on request), and I can relate that it was just like hitting a truck tire. The first time he asked me to hit him with full force, I was very reluctant to do so because I did not want to hurt him. However, after punching him a few times, it was obvious that the only thing that would get hurt was my hand and wrist. He was totally invulnerable to my punches. During sparring with his students he would alternate between being a truck tire and an elusive target against which no force could be applied.

Chen felt that it was important to be able to take punches because there are some situations in which neutralization is difficult, if not impossible (e.g., your back is against a wall). In class he once gave an account of a fight that was unavoidable and that he could not have won had he been unable to take punches without getting hurt. He was in a movie theater and asked a young man who was creating a disturbance to be quiet. The young man called his father, who then waited outside the movie theater for Chen. When Chen walked out, the father attacked him without warning. Chen told us, "I took a few punches, and then hit him in the jaw." (The punch was so hard that the jaw was broken in a number of places.) "Some people who saw the fight swore that I broke his jaw without touching him, using 'Ch'i at a distance.' But I know that I *did* hit him with my hand, because it hurt afterward." Chen frequently said, "If you want to be a good fighter, you'd better be able to take punches."

Professor Cheng did not advocate our "taking punches," although, on one occasion, he did allow one student, Khaleel Sayad, a third-degree Aikido practitioner, to hit him twice in the lower abdomen with full force. During impact, Cheng remained perfectly rooted and was totally unharmed.

Of course, Cheng's demonstration of his ability to stand firm against a powerful push or punch was not intended to imply that students should be solely developing standing firm as a basic method.

ATTITUDE

Investment in Loss

Cheng Man-ch'ing repeatedly emphasized the importance of "investing in loss." I interpreted this paradoxical expression to mean that, in order to progress at push-hands, the student must forego the use of improper techniques (impulsive maneuvers or rigid strength) to keep from being pushed or to uproot others.

The problem is that the principles of push-hands are so difficult to master that the student must spend considerable time (usually measured in years) attending to the principles alone. Thus, there is a long interval of time during which the student will not be able to evade being pushed and will be unable to properly uproot his partner. Even after considerable skill is achieved in rooting, neutralizing, receiving, and returning, the willingness to invest in loss is still required for continued progress. When a powerful opponent attacks with great force, there is a strong tendency to revert to the use of contractive muscular strength to avoid being pushed. Instead, it is crucial to use this opportunity to try to achieve a deeper state of sung. Thwarting the push by using contractive muscular force wastes an opportunity to learn and reinforces an improper response. Of course, there will be an initial period during which practitioners will get pushed frequently.

As previously stated, most of our learning experiences (in particular, schooling) have led us to become goal oriented. We are easily discouraged when we do not get an immediate result. In school, the first student to raise his or her hand is usually the first to be called upon and then praised if he has the correct answer. The rest of the students in the class may be learning at a good rate, but they tend to feel that the result—rather than the process—is what is paramount. This attitude, which many of us have accepted, sabotages the learning process.

Under Cheng Man-ch'ing I began to realize that practicing push-hands with the goal of uprooting my classmates as much as possible and being uprooted by my classmates as little as possible would stunt my growth. My allowing a classmate to execute a nice push when I was unable to neutralize accomplished a number of constructive things: (1) My classmate would have an opportunity to practice his or her push, (2) I would have an opportunity to experience a correctly executed push, (3) I would not falsely believe that, just because I thwarted a classmate's push, I had neutralized it, (4) a spirit of cooperation rather than competition would be fostered, and (5) egotistical impulses and goal orientation would be reduced.

During the time that I studied under Cheng, I occasionally paired off to do push-hands with an older brother,[5] Lou Kleinsmith. Lou was much more advanced than I and was continually able to uproot me. Occasionally, I got Lou off balance during a moment of his inattentiveness. My getting the better of him resulted in his repeatedly smashing me with great force into the wall. (Cheng was very concerned that students would be severely injured if pushed "into the room," and all pushing had to be done "into the wall." In fact, one student who owned a rug store graciously offered to cover the school walls, which were bare brick, with soft rugs, at his own expense. Cheng replied that it was very beneficial to our organs for us to hit the bare wall and declined the offer.)

Even though I accepted that it was good for my organs, I still had a substantial fear of hitting the wall. However, I soon learned how to withstand the impact comfortably and felt more secure with a wall behind me. Also, I realized that the less I tried to evade Lou's pushes, the softer they got. As time went on, I paired off with Lou at least once each practice session. He used this practice as an opportunity to refine his push, and I tried to discover exactly how he pushed me. I would concentrate on feeling how he contacted me and how he varied the pressure as the push built up. Little by little, my understanding increased, and I began to grasp the details of Lou's push.

William C. C. Chen also emphasized the attitude of "investing in loss." He had a beautiful way of getting his students to put this attitude into practice. He would say that, when encountering a partner's resistance while pushing him, you should stop and create an opportunity for him to relieve the resistance. If the partner is unable to use this opportunity, you should then try to show him how. Practice would then continue until either of the two partners encountered resistance in the other. Because this way of practicing understandably lacked a spirited quality and did not lead to any uprooting, it was not done continuously but as one of many exercises.

Feeding the Beginner

The beginner should be periodically given an opportunity to pair off with more experienced practitioners. The experienced one should be very careful not to push the beginner with such impact as to instill fear. The whole idea behind practice is to build a feeling of mutual trust and security, both of which conduce to relaxation and to cultivating the ability to observe movement and interpret force. When the element of fear pervades practice, the ensuing tension acts as a barrier to progress. The experienced practitioner should push the beginner gently until the beginner is not fearful of more aggressive pushes. Moreover, the experienced practitioner should allow himself to be pushed by the beginner and occasionally "set himself up" to give an opportunity to the beginner. For example, the experienced practitioner might aim his push, not to the beginner's center, but sufficiently off to the side that the beginner can neutralize it. Also, the experienced practitioner might purposely over-extend sufficiently so that the beginner can observe and take advantage of this error.

Cooperation and Sharing of Knowledge Versus Competition

The underlying concept of competition is that of comparing one's skill with or pitting it against that of others. According to this concept, he who can defeat another then feels satisfied that his efforts have borne fruit.

True accomplishment is relative to one's self—not others. Ideally the highest fulfillment occurs when you have made inner progress and when this fulfillment is independent of the accomplishments of others. If you truly seek to improve, you should seize an opportunity to do so even if, in the process, another is caused to improve to an even greater extent. Indeed, the devoted practitioner of any art eventually becomes a teacher and, in the process of doing so, lifts both himself and others.

Furthermore, if the art being taught is to continually evolve to higher and higher levels, each generation of students must surpass its teachers. It is selfish for a teacher to take without giving in return. Full giving by a teacher should result in his students progressing faster than he did. By being generous, the teacher also progresses at a faster rate than if he kept his skill from being learned by others.

In ancient China, a master of martial arts depended upon his knowledge for the preservation of his life. It was crucial that knowledge not be shared with a student until that student's trustworthiness was ascertained. Otherwise, the student might use the knowledge against the teacher or inadvertently expose what was learned to an enemy of the teacher. This danger has traditionally stood in the way of a teacher readily sharing his skills with any but his immediate family. In today's world, this kind of danger is essentially non-existent. Today there is an urgent need for people to learn a discipline such as T'ai Chi Ch'uan, which has so many spiritual and health benefits—especially in later years. Therefore, there is no compelling reason for a teacher to hide knowledge.

Freely sharing knowledge with others has two distinct advantages. By helping others to improve, you can contribute to the growth of the art and to the growth of others. Also, by sharing knowledge, you improve your own understanding as you attempt to teach others and are challenged by their questions.

To be considered a master by one's students makes it difficult to be seen acting in any manner beneath this level. There is a danger that teachers in this position can become stunted in their progress if they feel that they must hide limitations, errors, or faults from their students. Teachers of push-hands especially owe it both to themselves and their students *not to hide* their imperfections but to use them for mutual learning.

Notes

1. Cheng Man-ch'ing, *T'ai Chi Ch'uan: A Simplified Method of Calisthenics & Self Defense,* pp. 116–123.

2. See Cheng Man-ch'ing, *T'ai Chi Ch'uan: A Simplified Method of Calisthenics & Self Defense,* pp. 124–125.

3. *The Essence of T'ai-Chi Ch'uan: The Literary Tradition,* p. 57.

4. See Yearning K. Chen, *T'ai-Chi Ch'uan—Its Effects and Practical Applications,* Ohara Publications, Los Angeles, CA, (no date), p. 20.

5. A senior student is called an older brother.

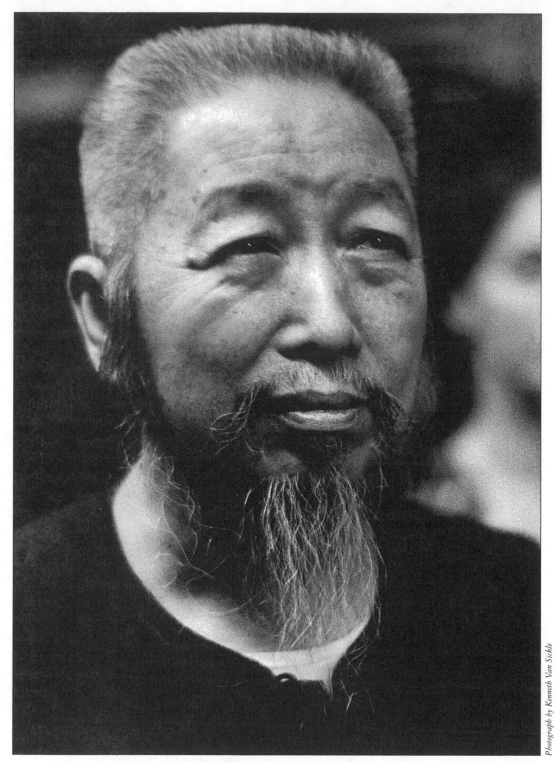

Cheng Man-ch'ing (1902-1975)

The Thirty-Seven Postures of Cheng Man-ch'ing's Short Form

Comments:

1. See chapter 7 for a discussion of the basic stances and for definitions of the terms referring to them.

2. All the figures showing the transitions and final postures are at the end of this Appendix.

NAMES OF POSTURES

1. Preparation
2. Beginning
3. Ward off with Left Hand
4. Ward off with Right Hand
5. Roll Back
6. Press
7. Push
8. Single Whip
9. Lift Hands
10. Strike with Shoulder
11. White Crane Spreads Wings
12. Brush Knee, Left
13. Hands Playing the P'i P'a
14. Step Forward, Deflect Downward, and Punch
15. Withdraw and Push
16. Cross Hands
17. Embrace Tiger, Return to Mountain
18. Looking at Fist Under Elbow
19. Step Back to Repulse Monkey, Right Side

20. Step Back to Repulse Monkey, Left Side
21. Diagonal Flying
22. Cloud Hands, Left
23. Cloud Hands, Right
24. Descending Single Whip
25. Golden Cock Stands on One Leg, Right Side
26. Golden Cock Stands on One Leg, Left Side
27. Separate Right Foot
28. Separate Left Foot
29. Turn and Kick with Heel
30. Brush Knee, Right
31. Step Forward and Strike Downward
32. The Fairy Weaving at the Shuttle (NE)
33. The Fairy Weaving at the Shuttle (NW)
34. Step Forward to the Seven Stars of the Big Dipper
35. Step Back to Ride the Tiger
36. Turn the Body to Sweep the Lotus
37. Bend the Bow to Shoot the Tiger

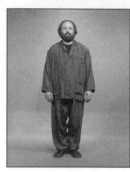

Fig. A-1

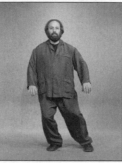

Fig. A-2

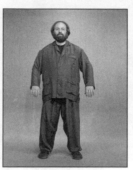

Fig. A-3

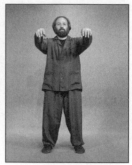

Fig. A-4

DESCRIPTION OF THE MOVEMENTS

1. Preparation

Stand facing north[1] with heels together and arms hanging at the sides (Fig. A-1). Lower the body by shifting the weight 100% onto the right foot. At the same time, the arms become alive and slightly bent at the elbows, and the hands rotate so that both palms face the rear. Next, step sideways with the left foot so that the heel moves directly west a distance of one shoulder width. In doing so, turn the body slightly to the right, rotating the left foot inward so that when it touches the ground, the center line of the left foot lies on a north-south line (Fig. A-2). Next, shift the weight to the left foot. Then turn the body slightly to the left, pivoting the right foot inward on the heel until its center line also lies on a north-south line. Next, shift the weight 50% onto the right foot, and at the same time, come up to standing with the knees straight but not locked. The palms of the hands face the rear, elbows slightly bent, and the thumbs are at the centers of the sides of the thighs. Both feet should be parallel, pointing north, and a shoulder width apart. Both heels should lie on an east-west line (Fig. A-3).

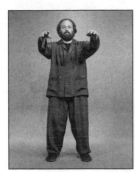
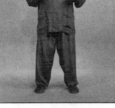
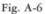
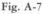
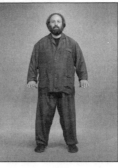
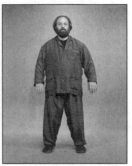

| Fig. A-5 | Fig. A-6 | Fig. A-7 | Fig. A-8 |

2. Beginning

Keeping the knees straight but loose, lift both arms until the tops of the wrists are at shoulder level. The hands, elbows, and shoulders droop. The elbows are slightly bent. When the wrists reach shoulder level, they stop (Fig. A-4). Next, the hands continue to rotate upward until they are parallel to the floor, with the middle finger of each hand pointing forward (Fig. A-5). Next, the elbows bend and lower, so that the wrists move toward the body and slightly downward until the elbows are slightly behind the back, and the tops of the wrists are at armpit level. While the wrists are moving inward, they flex, so that the hands remain parallel to the floor, and the middle fingers continue to point directly forward (Fig. A-6). Next, the wrists lower and flex, so that the fingers now point slightly upward. When the wrists reach their lowest position, with elbows slightly bent (Fig. A-7), the hands then rotate downward until the wrists are in their centered positions. The palm of each hand faces rearward with the thumb midway between the front and back of the thigh (Fig. A-8).

Comments: See chapter 7 for a discussion of the fifty-fifty stance with straight knees.

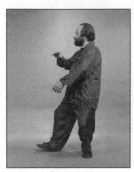
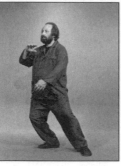
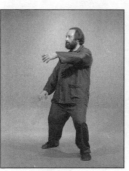
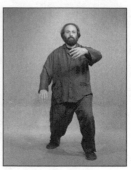

Fig. A-9   Fig. A-10   Fig. A-11   Fig. A-12

3. Ward off with Left Hand

Shift the weight 100% onto the left foot, and simultaneously turn the body to the right. At the same time, the right foot pivots on its heel to point eastward, and the hands move to a position of holding a large ball in front of the center of the chest, with the right hand above, the left hand below, and both palms facing each other (Fig. A-9). Then shift the weight 100% onto the right foot. While you are shifting the weight, the left heel rises slightly off the ground in preparation for a step. Next, turn your body slightly to the left. At the same time, step northward with the left foot, keeping the shoulder width of the previous posture (Fig. A-10). Next, the weight shifts 70% onto the left foot, so that the knee reaches a vertical line through the tip of the middle toe of the left foot (Fig. A-11). Next, turn the body to face north, simultaneously pivoting the right foot on its heel to point northeastward. At the same time, the left hand circles to a position in front of the center of the chest, palm facing inward, and the right hand moves vertically down, ending up with the palm facing the rear near the right thigh (Fig. A-12).

Comments: This is a 70-30 position facing north (see chapter 7). One of the most common errors is that of losing the width of the stance during stepping. It is essential that the left foot step northward without arcing toward the east.

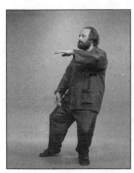
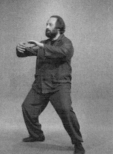
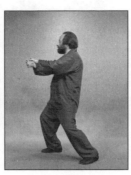
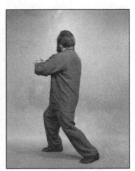

| Fig. A-13 | Fig. A-14 | Fig. A-15 | Fig. A-16 |

4. Ward off with Right Hand

Shift the weight 100% onto the left foot, turning the body slightly to the right. At the same time, the right foot pivots to the right on its ball, and the hands move to a position of holding a large ball in front of the center of the chest, with the left hand above, the right hand below, and both palms facing each other (Fig. A-13). Next, step eastward with the right foot, possibly making a correction to provide a shoulder width. Next, shift the weight 70% onto the right foot, so that the right knee reaches a vertical line through the tip of the middle toe of the right foot (Fig. A-14). Next, turn the body to face east, simultaneously pivoting the left foot on its heel to the northeast. At the same time, the right hand rises to a position in front of the center of the chest, palm facing inward. The left hand does not move with respect to the body, thus ending up in front of the center of the chest with the palm facing downward and the fingers pointing toward the palm of the right hand (Fig. A-15).

Comments. The ch'i travels through the left forearm, out of the hollow of the left hand, into the hollow of the right hand, and down the right forearm.

5. Roll Back

Turn the body to the southeast, keeping the weight 70% on the right foot. The right knee does not move during the turning, and the hands do not move appreciably with respect to the body (Fig. A-16). Next, without turning left, shift the weight 100% onto the left foot. At the same time, the right hand rises to the height of the mouth, the left hand lowers and rotates to a palm-up position under the right elbow (Fig. A-17). Then the body turns to the north (Fig. A-18).

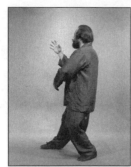

Fig. A-17

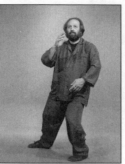

Fig. A-18

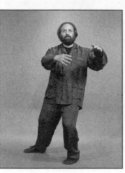

Fig. A-19

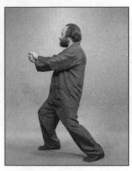

Fig. A-20

6. Press

Continuing, the left hand circles downward toward the left thigh, and then upward to the height of the shoulder (Fig. A-19). Next, shift the weight 70% onto the right foot, and then turn the body to the right to face east. The hands end up touching each other as follows: The right hand is in front of the center of the chest, with the palm facing slightly upward. The heel of the left hand nestles in the center of the right hand, and the thumb heel of the right hand nestles in the center of the left hand. The thumb of the right hand, and the little finger of the left hand form the letter V (Fig. A-20).

Comments. The nestling of the heels and hollows of the hands resembles the interlacing of the yin and yang shapes of the T'ai Chi symbol.

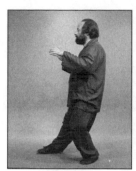 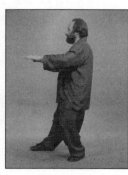 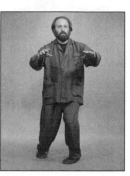

| Fig. A-21 | Fig. A-22 | Fig. A-23 | Fig. A-24 |

7. Push

Shift the weight back 100% onto the left foot, letting the hands naturally separate, so that the palms are facing forward and slightly downward (Fig. A-21). Next shift forward into a 70-30 position, the hands moving with the body (Fig. A-22).

Comments: A good image is that of pushing a heavy object, such as an upright piano. If the arms alone are used, the person pushing will be moved backward, whereas if the body is used the push will be more successful.

8. Single Whip

Shift the weight 100% onto the left foot, simultaneously lowering both hands to mid chest and in front of the body (Fig. A-23). Next, rotate the body 90° to the left. At the same time, pivot the right foot on its heel to point northward. The hands move horizontally with the body, with one hand on each side of the medial plane (Fig. A-24). Next, shift the weight 100% onto the right foot. At the same time, the left hand lowers to a position in front of the pubic region, the right hand circles counterclockwise in a horizontal plane close to the center of the chest, forming a bird's beak (all the fingers touch the thumb, and the hand hangs from the wrist, which is at shoulder level) (Fig. A-25). Next, turn the body to the northeast, keeping the weight 100% on the right foot. Next, still keeping the weight 100% on the right foot, turn the body to the northwest while pivoting on the ball of the left foot. At the same time, the bird's beak moves outward from the body and the left hand rises to armpit level (Fig. A-26). Next, the left foot steps into what will become a 70-30 stance facing west. Then shift the weight 70% onto the left foot. At the same time, the left hand moves to a position in front of the face, palm inward and fingers upward. Next, while turning the body to face west, the left hand turns outward and the right foot pivots inward on the heel. The left hand ends up in front of the left shoulder (Fig. A-27).

Comments: The two most common errors are moving the hands on their own and shifting the weight to the right during the initial turning to the left.

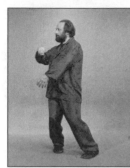
Fig. A-25

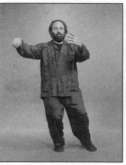
Fig. A-26

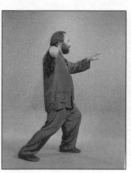
Fig. A-27

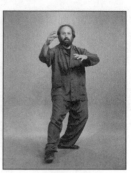
Fig. A-28

9. Lift Hands

Shift the weight 100% onto the left foot. At the same time, the body turns to the right and the bird's beak opens. Then, the hands come together as the body turns to the left until it points northwest. At the same time, the right foot moves to a position with the heel touching the floor on the north-south line of the heel of the left foot. The head and hands point north. The left hand is opposite the right elbow, and the fingertips of the right hand are at neck level (Fig. A-28).

Comments: This is the first posture with 100% of the weight on one foot.

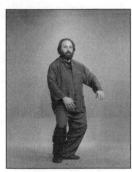
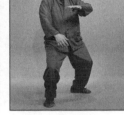
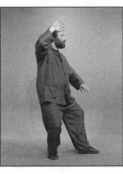
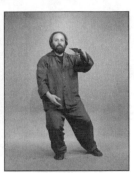

| Fig. A-29 | Fig. A-30 | Fig. A-31 | Fig. A-32 |

10. Strike with Shoulder

Keeping the weight 100% on the left foot, lower the left hand to a position just outside the left thigh and lower the right hand to a position in front of the pubic area. At the same time, the arch of the right foot is brought next to the heel of the left foot (Fig. A-29). Next, the right foot steps forward and slightly to the right in order to achieve a stable width. Next, the left hand circles to a position near the right elbow, fingers pointing forward. The direction of the head and right forearm is north. The body faces northwest but the head faces northward (Fig. A-30).

Comments: This is a 70-30 posture.

11. White Crane Spreads Wings

Shift the weight 100% onto the right foot. At the same time, the body turns slightly to the left, the right hand rises and rotates to a palm-out position near the right temple, the left hand lowers to a palm-slightly-out position just outside the left thigh, and the ball of the left foot moves to a position touching an east-west line passing through the heel of the right foot. The head faces west, and the body faces northwest (Fig. A-31).

Comments: Professor Cheng emphasized that all the body parts arrive at their final positions simultaneously.

12. Brush Knee, Left

The right hand lowers in a circular movement in the medial plane and simultaneously turns palm up just outside the right thigh. Next, keeping the weight 100% on the right foot, turn the body to the right, pivoting on the ball of the left foot. At the same time, the left hand circles, palm down, upward and to the right (Fig. A-32). Next, turn slightly to the left, keeping the weight 100% on the right leg. At the same time the right hand rises to the level of the mouth and the left hand lowers to a level just below the navel (Fig. A-33). This initial turning of the body to the left initiates a step into a 70-30 position with the left foot. Next, shift the weight 70% onto the left foot, and turn the body to face west. At the same time, the right hand moves forward past the mouth to a position in front of the

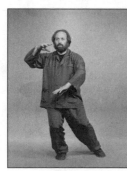
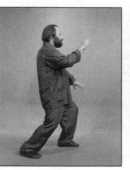
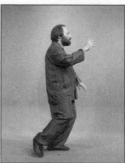
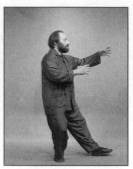

Fig. A-33   Fig. A-34   Fig. A-35   Fig. A-36

right shoulder, the left hand circles laterally to a position to the left of the left thigh, and the right foot pivots on its heel until it points northwest (Fig. A-34).

13. Hands Playing the P'i P'a

Without rising upward, shift the weight 100% onto the left foot, lifting the right foot slightly off the ground (Fig. A-35). Next, step back onto the right foot. As the weight shifts 100% onto the right foot, the left hand circles clockwise and away from the body to chin level. At the same time, the right hand lowers to a position near the left elbow, and the left foot moves to a position with the heel touching the floor on an east-west line passing through the heel of the right foot. The body faces northwest, and the hands and head point west (Fig. A-36).

Comments: This posture is essentially the opposite side of "Raise Hands." The p'i p'a is a fretted four-string instrument resembling a lute.

Brush Knee, Left. This posture is the same as (12), except that the initial turning involves a pivot on the heel of the left foot (Figs. A-32 through A-34).

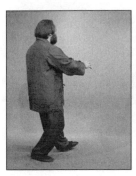

Fig. A-37

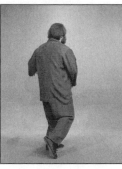

Fig. A-38

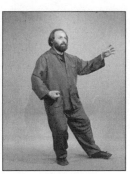

Fig. A-39

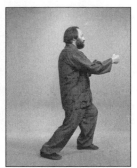

Fig. A-40

14. Step Forward, Deflect Downward, and Punch

Shift the weight 100% onto the right foot, and, at the same time, turn the body to the southwest and pivot the left foot on its heel until it points southwest. At the same time, the hands lower slightly (Fig. A-37). Next, shift the weight 100% onto the left foot, simultaneously lowering the right hand near the left thigh. A "hollow" fist is formed with the right hand just as it reaches its lowest position (Fig. A-38). Next, the body turns to the right, initiating a short semicircular "crescent" step to the northwest with the right foot. As the weight shifts 100% onto the right foot, the body turns to the northwest. At the same time, (a) the right fist circles upward to the level of the chin and down outside the right thigh, with the knuckles downward; and (b) the left hand rises, turning palm out as it passes near the left ear, and then it extends forward, rotating so that the palm faces north. Next, the left foot steps forward into what will become a 70-30 stance in the westerly direction (Fig. A-39). Then, shift the weight 70% onto the left foot. At the same time, the right fist rises to waist level. Then, the body turns to face west, simultaneously extending the fist outward and rotating it into a vertical position. At the same time, the left hand moves slightly inward to a position above and to the left of the right forearm (Fig. A-40).

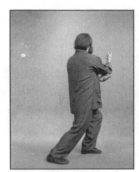

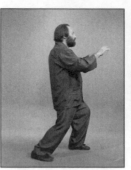

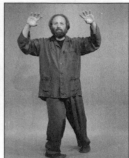

Fig. A-41   Fig. A-42   Fig. A-43   Fig. A-44

15. Withdraw and Push

Turn the body to the southwest, keeping the weight 70% on the left foot. The left knee does not move during the turning. At the same time, the fist extends and crosses the center line of the body, while the left hand crosses the center of the body to come palm up under the right triceps (Fig. A-41). Next, shift the weight 100% onto the right foot, and turn the body to the right. During the turning and shifting of the body, the right elbow makes a counter clockwise circle around the left palm in a horizontal plane. As the elbows move rearward, the hands come in front of the chest, palms facing inward (Fig. A-42). Next, the body shifts forward until 70% of the weight is on the left foot and then turns to face west. At the same time, the hands rotate until the palms face forward (Fig. A-43).

16. Cross Hands

Shift the weight 100% onto the right foot, and turn to face north. At the same time, the hands move with the body and also slightly upward. The left foot pivots on the heel and turns with the body to point north (Fig. A-44). Next, shift the weight 100% onto the left foot, simultaneously bringing the hands outward and downward in a large circle in vertical plane in the east-west direction. At the same time, the right foot pivots inward on its ball until it points north. If the previous 70-30 stance was correct, the feet should be a shoulder width apart, with the right foot slightly ahead of the left foot (Fig. A-45). When the hands reach the bottom of the circle, bring the right foot to the same feet-parallel stance as the "Beginning" posture. Next, shift the weight 50% onto the right foot, simul- taneously raising the hands to a crossed position in front of the center of the chest. The left hand is on top. The palms face inward, and the wrist joints nestle one into the other (Fig. A-46).

Comments: Professor Cheng regarded the learning of the movements up to this point as a "substantial beginning." He said that this first section contained most of the basic types of movements contained in the entire form. The "Cross Hands" posture is done with the weight equally divided between both feet. This

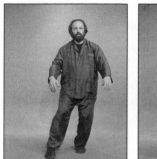

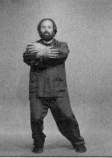

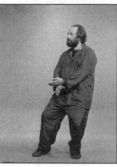

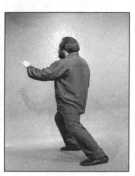

| Fig. A-45 | Fig. A-46 | Fig. A-47 | Fig. A-48 |

weighting is not considered to be an error since the posture in question is more of a meditative/Ch'i Kung stance than a fighting stance.

17. Embrace Tiger, Return to Mountain

Shift the weight 100% onto the left foot, simultaneously turning slightly to the right and lowering the hands, back to back (Fig. A-47). The wrists remain in contact. Turn to the right, and step southeast with the right foot. The right hand moves with the body, whereas the left hand rises to about mouth level. Then the weight shifts 70% onto the right foot. Next, the body turns to face southeast, simultaneously pivoting the left foot on the heel to point east, and striking forward with the left hand. At the same time, the right hand rotates to a palm-up position outside the right thigh. This is a diagonal 70-30 position similar to "Brush Knee" (Fig. A-48). Then repeat postures 5, 6, 7, and 8, (Figs. A-17 through A-27), oriented diagonally. "Diagonal Single Whip" is shown in Fig. A-49.

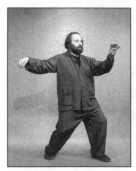 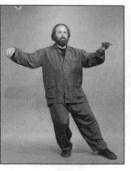 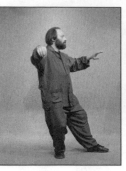 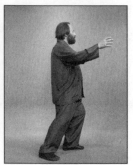

Fig. A-49   Fig. A-50   Fig. A-51   Fig. A-52

18. Looking at Fist Under Elbow

Shift the weight 100% onto the right foot. At the same time, the left hand extends outward to about neck level (Fig. A-50). Next, turn the body until the left foot, which becomes airborne and moves with the body, points west (Fig. A-51). Then shift the weight 100% onto the left foot, simultaneously opening the bird's beak of the previous posture (Fig. A-52). Until the end of this posture, the right hand remains at essentially the same level in the medial plane, thus moving with the body. Continue turning to the left, and place the right foot so that its ball is on the same north-south line as the heel of the left foot. The right foot now points northwest. Then shift the weight 100% onto the right foot and turn the body to point southwest (Fig. A-53). Next, keeping the weight 100% on the right foot, turn to the right. At the same time, the left hand thrusts forward and upward with the turning of the body. The palm of the left hand faces north. The right hand, which, until now, has remained in the medial plane at neck level, lowers and forms a vertical fist below the left elbow (Fig. A-54).

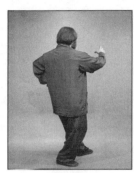
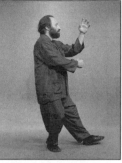
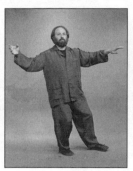
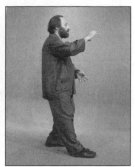

| Fig. A-53 | Fig. A-54 | Fig. A-55 | Fig. A-56 |

19. Step Back to Repulse Monkey, Right Side

Keeping the weight 100% on the right foot, turn to the right. At the same time, the fist of the previous posture releases, the right hand makes a large circle, palm up past the right thigh, and up to mouth level, palm up. Additionally, the left hand extends westward at throat level, palm down, and the left foot pivots with the body on its heel (Fig. A-55). Then, the body turns slightly to the left, initiating a step eastward with the left foot. At the same time, the palm of the right hand rotates to face downward. The left foot steps, toe first, on an east-west line a shoulder width south of the right heel. As the weight shifts back, the body points toward the northwest, and the hands do not move relative to the body. After the weight has completely shifted, the body turns to point west, and, simultaneously, the right foot pivots on its heel to point west. At the same time, the left hand lowers to a position, palm up near the left thigh, and the right hand moves to a position in front of the right shoulder, palm forward (Fig. A-56).

Comments: Professor Cheng emphasized the importance of the following: The parallelism of the feet, maintaining a shoulder width, finishing of the posture by turning into square instead of over-turning, the connection of the hands through the center of the body, and that the palms of the two hands always are opposite to each other. Cheng repeatedly said that pointing the toes outward prevents the ch'i from passing through the weilu "gate" in the region of the sacrum. This gate is considered to be an important opening through which ch'i enters the body.

From the point of view of coordination, "Step Back to Repulse Monkey" probably is the most difficult movement in the form to do properly. It may take quite a long time before stepping back with feet parallel feels natural.

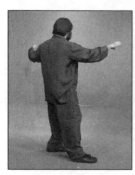

Fig. A-57

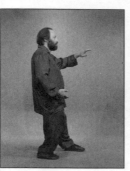

Fig. A-58

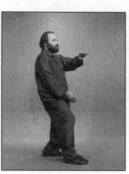

Fig. A-59

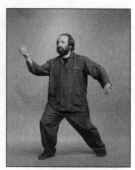

Fig. A-60

20. Step Back to Repulse Monkey, Left Side

Turn to the left. At the same time extend the right hand and rotate it palm downward (Fig. A-57). Then, turn slightly to the right, simultaneously rotating both hands, right palm up and left palm down. Step back with the right foot, and turn to face west. The weight is 100% on the right foot (Fig. A-58).

Comments: Any even number of alternate-sided repetitions may be done. Although doing the four repetitions listed is standard, doing only two repetitions is useful where a space or time limitation is a problem.

21. Diagonal Flying

The last "Repulse Monkey" will end with the weight 100% on the left foot. Then, turn the body to the left, circling the hands clockwise on the left side of the body, until they seem to hold a large ball. The left hand is above, palm down, and the right hand is below, palm up. Then the body turns to the right (Fig. A-59). The turning of the body initiates a step with the right foot in the northeast direction. After the weight shifts 70% onto the right leg, the body turns to point to the northeast. At the same time, the left foot pivots on the heel to point north, and the hands separate. The right hand ends up palm up, at about throat level, and the left hand is palm down near the left thigh. This is a diagonal-70-30 posture (Fig. A-60).

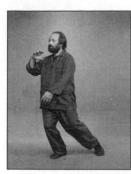

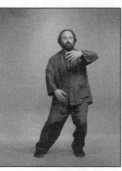

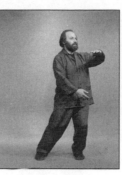

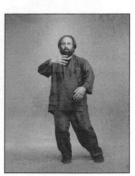

| Fig. A-61 | Fig. A-62 | Fig. A-63 | Fig. A-64 |

22. Cloud Hands, Left

Shift the weight 100% onto the right foot, simultaneously turning to the right and rotating the hands with palms facing each other as if holding a large ball (Fig. A-61). The turning initiates a small step northward with the left foot so that the heels of both feet are on the same east-west line. The left foot points north. Then shift the weight 100% onto the left foot, simultaneously lowering the right hand to the level of the pubic region. Then turn the body to the left, simultaneously pivoting the right foot to point north (feet parallel). At the same time, the left hand rises to neck level. When the body points north the hands are in the medial plane, palms facing the body (Fig. A-62). When the body is fully turned to the left, the palms face each other, left hand on top, still in the medial plane. The right foot is empty (Fig. A-63).

Comments: Professor Cheng cautioned against bending the wrists during the transitions. He repeatedly emphasized that the two hands should remain in the medial plane throughout.

23. Cloud Hands, Right

The last part of the turning in the previous movement initiates a step to the left of the right foot, which moves along an east-west line to a position where the center lines of the feet lie along north-south lines one-half shoulder width apart. Shift the weight 100% onto the right foot, simultaneously lowering the left hand and then raising the right hand. Then turn to the right. When the body points north the hands are in the medial plane, palms facing the body (Fig. A-64). When the body is fully turned to the right, the palms face each other, right hand on top, still in the medial plane. The left foot is empty (Fig. A-65).

Cloud Hands, Left, Right, and Left. Repeat postures 22, 23, and 22, respectively.

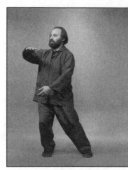
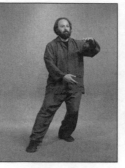
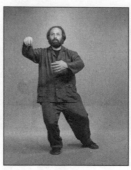
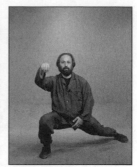

| Fig. A-65 | Fig. A-66 | Fig. A-67 | Fig. A-68 |

Single Whip. After the last "Cloud Hands," the weight is 100% on the left foot. The final turning of the body to the left initiates a step with the right foot northward (Fig. A-66). Then shift the weight 100% onto the right, and turn slightly to the left, pivoting on the ball of the left foot. At the same time, the hands circle downward and then out toward the right. The right hand forms the familiar "bird's beak" (Fig. A-67). Then the left foot steps into what will become a 70-30 stance. As the weight shifts 70% onto the left foot the left hand circles up near the right armpit. Then as the body turns, the left hand turns outward, as in the previous "Single Whip" (Fig. A-27).

24. Descending Single Whip

Turn the body to face north, simultaneously pivoting the right foot on its heel to point north. At the same time, the left hand circles clockwise to a position in front of the pubic region, pointing inward. Keeping the weight 100% on the right foot, lower the body to a squatting position. The right heel does not lift off the floor, and the right hand remains extended in the bird's-beak fist (Fig. A-68). Then turn the body to the left, simultaneously pivoting the left foot to the south-west on its heel and turning the right hand palm out (Fig. A-69). Next, shift the weight 70% onto the left foot, simultaneously raising the left hand to face level (Fig. A-70).

Comments: It is essential that a correct alignment of the spine and pelvis be maintained while doing this movement. Maintaining correct alignment will limit the degree to which you will be able to descend. However, it will be found that keeping a correct alignment will result in a highly beneficial opening of the thigh joints.

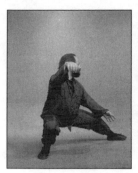 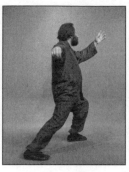 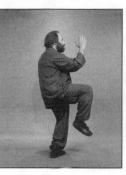 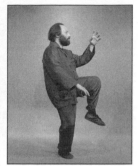

Fig. A-69   Fig. A-70   Fig. A-71   Fig. A-72

25. Golden Cock Stands on One Leg, Right Side

Shift the weight 100% onto the left leg, simultaneously extending the left hand forward to the level of the mouth. Next, come up to a sitting position on the left foot. At the same time, the left hand lowers to a position just outside the left thigh, the right knee rises to waist level, and the right hand rises to the level of the mouth, palm facing south (Fig. A-71).

Comments: The right foot hangs from the knee in a relaxed, natural manner.

26. Golden Cock Stands on One Leg, Left Side

Step to the northeast with the right foot. Next, shift the weight 100% onto the right foot. At the same time, the right hand lowers to a position just outside the right thigh, the left knee rises to waist level, and the left hand rises to the level of the mouth, palm facing north (Fig. A-72).

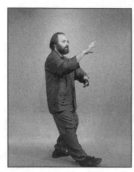
Fig. A-73

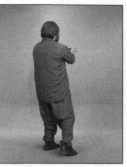
Fig. A-74

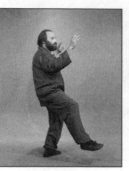
Fig. A-75

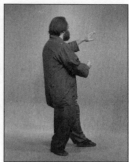
Fig. A-76

27. Separate Right Foot

Step to the southeast with the left foot. Next, shift the weight 100% onto the left foot. At the same time, the right hand moves to a palm-down position near the left elbow, and the left hand lowers and extends slightly. Then turn the body to face northwest, simultaneously pivoting the right foot outward on its heel to turn with the body. At the same time, the right hand extends outward, and the left hand moves to a palm-up position near the right elbow (Fig. A-73). The hands stay in the medial plane. Then, keeping the weight 100% on the left foot, turn the body to the south, simultaneously lowering both hands together, palms facing each other. At the same time, the right foot pivots inward on its heel to turn with the body. Next, turn the body to the southwest, simultaneously lifting both hands to a wrists-touching position in front of the face. The palms face inward, and the left wrist is above the right wrist (Fig. A-74). Then, continue to turn until the body points west. At the same time, the hands turn outward, the right hand extends forward, and the right foot pivots outward on its ball and then kicks to the northwest at about knee level (Fig. A-75).

28. Separate Left Foot

Release the right knee, so that the lower part of the right leg naturally swings inward and then back out. Shift the weight 100% onto the right foot. Then, turn the body to the left, circling the hands so that the left hand is extended, palm down, and the right hand is palm up below the left elbow. At the same time, the left foot steps inward and touches on its ball (Fig. A-76). Next, turn the body to the north, simultaneously lowering both hands together, palms facing each other. Next, turn the body to the northwest, simultaneously lifting both hands to a wrists-touching position in front of the face. The palms face inward, and the right wrist is above the left wrist (Fig. A-77). Then, continue to turn until the body points west. At the same time, the hands turn outward, the left hand extends forward, and the left foot kicks to the southwest at about knee level (Fig. A-78).

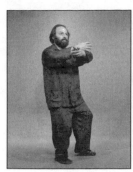
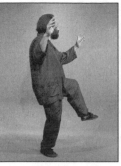
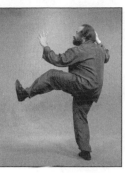
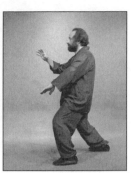

Fig. A-77   Fig. A-78   Fig. A-79   Fig. A-80

29. Turn and Kick with Heel

From the previous posture, raise the left knee to waist level, and turn the body to the right. The right knee does not buckle outward, and the left leg does not move relative to the body. The action is as though a spring in the right thigh joint were being compressed. Next, release the "spring," and allow the body to turn to the left, pivoting on the heel of the right foot. When the right foot points south, the ball of the right foot is lowered, and the hands cross in front of the neck, palms inward and right hand on the outside. Next, the body continues to turn, simultaneously lifting the left knee and kicking to the east with the left heel. At the same time, the hands separate and turn kicks outward. The left hand also extends eastward (Fig. A-79). Then step into "Brush Knee, Left" (Fig. A-80).

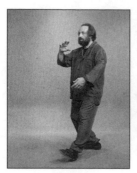

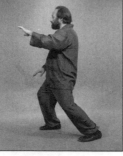

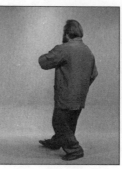

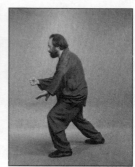

| Fig. A-81 | Fig. A-82 | Fig. A-83 | Fig. A-84 |

30. Brush Knee, Right

Shift the weight 100% onto the right foot, and turn to the left, simultaneously pivoting the left foot on its heel to point northeast. At the same time, the right hand moves with the body, at mouth level, and the left hand rotates to palm up, so that both hands are as if holding a large ball (Fig. A-81). Then, without turning the body, shift the weight 100% onto the left foot. At the same time the left hand rises to a palm-down position near the mouth, and the right hand lowers to a palm-down position in front of the pubic region. Next, step eastward with the right foot into what will become a 70-30 position, and shift the weight 70% onto the right foot. Then turn the body to face east, simultaneously extending the left hand in front of the left shoulder and circling the right hand laterally to a position to the right of the right thigh (Fig. A-82).

31. Step Forward and Strike Downward

Shift the weight 100% onto the left foot, and turn to the right, simultaneously pivoting the right foot on its heel to point southeast. At the same time, the left hand moves with the body, at mouth level, and the right hand rotates to palm up, so that both hands are as if holding a large ball (Fig. A-83). Then, without turning the body, shift the weight 100% onto the right foot. At the same time the right hand forms a fist near the right thigh, and the left hand lowers to a palm-down position over the fist. Next, step into what will become a 70-30 position with the left foot, and shift the weight 70% onto the left foot. Then turn the body to face east, simultaneously extending and rotating the fist into a vertical orientation. At the same time, the left hand circles laterally to a position to the left of the left thigh (Fig. A-84).

Ward off with Right Hand, Rollback, Press, Withdraw and Push, and Single Whip. Next, shift the weight 100% on the right foot, simultaneously turning the left foot to the northeast. At the same the left hand rises to chest level, palm down. Then shift the weight 100% onto the left foot, simultaneously releasing the right fist. Next, step eastward with the right foot into a 70-30 stance. At

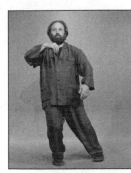
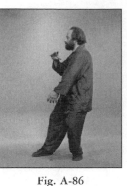
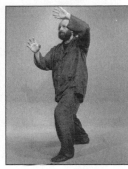
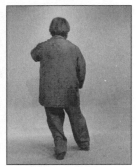

| Fig. A-85 | Fig. A-86 | Fig. A-87 | Fig. A-88 |

the same time the right hand rises to the "Ward off" posture (Fig. A-12). Then repeat postures 5–8 (Figs. A-13 through A-27).

32. The Fairy Weaving at the Shuttle (Northeast)

Shift the weight 100% onto the right foot, simultaneously circling the left hand downward. Then turn the body to point north, simultaneously pivoting on the heel of the left foot until its centerline lies along a north-south line (Fig. A-85). Shift the weight back 100% onto the left foot, simultaneously releasing the bird's beak of the previous posture and moving the right hand to a palm-down position in front of the center of the chest. Then turn the body to the right until the suspended right foot, which moves with the body, points east. Next, shift the weight 100% onto the right foot, and take a step with the left foot into what will become a 70-30 position facing northeast (Fig. A-86). As the weight shifts onto the left foot, the left hand rises to a position in front of the center of the forehead, palm facing inward. As the body turns to the northeast, (a) the right foot pivots to point east, (b) the palm of the left hand rotates outward, and (c) as a result of the turning, the right hand strikes outward with its fingertips about nose level (Fig. A-87).

Comments: This is the first of four moves also known as the "Four Corners."

33. The Fairy Weaving at the Shuttle (Northwest)

Shift the weight 100% onto the right foot, simultaneously lowering both hands slightly and turning the palms to face each other. Then turn the body to the south, simultaneously pivoting the left foot on its heel to point southward. Next, shift the weight 100% onto the left foot (Fig. A-88). Then turn the body to point westward, and step to the northwest into a 70-30 stance with the right foot. As the weight shifts 70% onto the right foot, the right hand rises to the level of the forehead, palm inward. Then turn the body to point northeast. At the same time, the right hand rotates palm out, the left hand extends about mouth level, and the left foot pivots on the heel to point westward (Fig. A-89).

Comments: If posture 32 ends with both heels almost on a north-south line, it will be difficult to execute posture 33. Instead, posture 32 should end with the

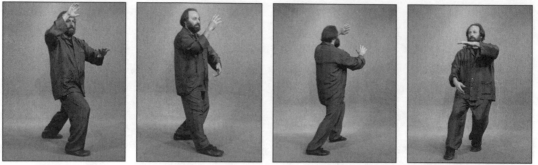

| Fig. A-89 | Fig. A-90 | Fig. A-91 | Fig. A-92 |

heel of the left foot almost one shoe length eastward of the north-south line through the heel of the left foot.

The Fairy Weaving at the Shuttle (Southwest). Shift the weight 100% onto the left foot (Fig. A-90), and side-step to the left with the right foot. Then take a step with the left foot to the southwest into posture 32 (Fig. A-91).

The Fairy Weaving at the Shuttle (Southeast). Except for orientation in space, the transition to this posture is the same as "The Fairy Weaving at the Shuttle (Northwest)" (Figs. A-92 through A-93).

Ward off with Left Hand, Ward off with Right Hand, Rollback, Press, Withdraw and Push, Single Whip, and Descending Single Whip. Shift the weight 100% onto the right foot, simultaneously lowering both hands into a "ball-holding" position (Fig. A-94). Then turn to the left and step into "Ward off Left" (posture 3) facing the north. Then repeat postures 4–8 and 24.

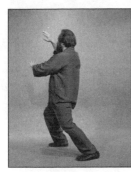 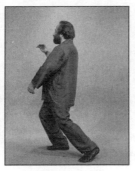 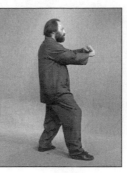 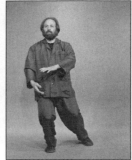

Fig. A-93   Fig. A-94   Fig. A-95   Fig. A-96

34. Step Forward to the Seven Stars (of the Big Dipper)

The left foot turns to point southwest, and then the weight shifts 100% onto the left foot with the ball of the right foot just touching an east-west line through the heel of the left foot. At the same time, both hands form fists which rise to a crossed position in front of the upper chest. The left fist is above, and the wrists nestle, one into the other (Fig. A-95).

35. Step Back to Ride the Tiger

Turn the body slightly to the right, and take a step to the northeast with the right foot pointed to the north. Shift the weight 100% onto the right foot, simultaneously opening the fists and rotating the hands so that the inside of the wrists touch. Turn the body to face north, at the same time circling both hands in front of the pubic region (Fig. A-96). Next the hands separate, and the right hand circles up to forehead level, palm facing forward. The left hand remains in front of the pubic region, palm inward. Next the body turns to the left, bringing the right hand forward near the ear and brushing the left hand across the left thigh to the outside (Fig. A-97). The final posture is similar to "White Crane Spreads Wings," except that the palm of the right hand faces forward, rather than to the side.

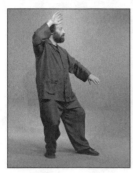
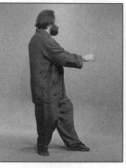
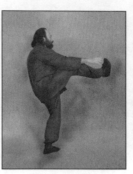
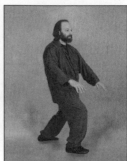

Fig. A-97   Fig. A-98   Fig. A-99   Fig. A-100

36. Turn the Body to Sweep the Lotus

Keeping the weight 100% on the right foot, turn the body to the left, stretching a "spring" in the right thigh joint but not moving the right knee. At the same time, the right hand lowers to a position in front of and facing the pubic region (Fig. A-98). Next, release the spring and turn to the right, pivoting on the ball of the right foot. When the left heel reaches an east-west line through the ball of the right foot, it touches down, and pivots to point southwest. At the same time, the weight begins to shift 100% onto the left foot, and the hands extend outward at mid-chest level from the centrifugal effect. Once the weight is 100% on the left foot, the right knee rises, such that this, combined with the continued turning of the body, brings the right foot upward in a clockwise circle. The toes of the right foot successively touch the left and right hands, both of which are now moving to the left (Fig. A-99). Then the right foot lowers to a position close to the knee of the left foot.

37. Bend the Bow to Shoot the Tiger

Continuing from the previous posture, the hands lower, the right foot steps to the northwest, and the weight shifts 70% onto the right foot (Fig. A-100). Next, the body turns to the right, and simultaneously the hands circle counterclockwise. Then the body turns to the left, and simultaneously, the hands form fists. The knuckles of the right hand face the right temple, and the axis of the left forearm is along a horizontal southwest line. The left fist is rotated to a position such that the line from the eyes to the fist parallels that of its hollow. Next turn the body slightly to the right, simultaneously extending the left fist in the southwest direction (Fig. A-101).

Step Forward, Deflect Downward, and Punch; Withdraw and Push; and Cross Hands. Shift the weight 100% onto the right foot, simultaneously opening the left fist (Fig. A-102). Next, lift the left foot and then place it back down in a comfortable orientation and position. Shift the weight 100% onto the left foot, simultaneously opening the right fist. Then turn to the left, pivoting on the heel of the right foot

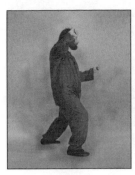

Fig. A-101

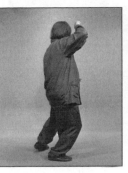

Fig. A-102

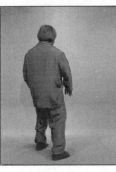

Fig. A-103

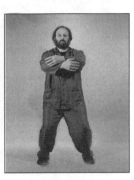

Fig. A-104

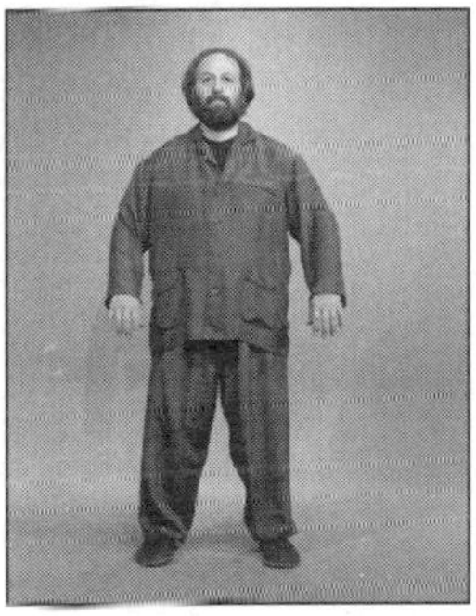

(Fig. A-103). Next, keeping the weight 100% on the left foot, turn to the right, pivoting on the ball of the right foot. At the same time, form a fist with the right hand. Then take a "crescent" step with the right foot, continuing into the "Punch," posture as described in 14. Then repeat postures 15 and 16, the latter with the knees bent and the weight equally distributed between both feet (Fig. A-104). End the form by coming up to standing, simultaneously lowering the hands as they naturally separate. The hands face the rear, thumbs at mid-thigh (Fig. A-105).

Comments: Professor Cheng emphasized to us that after the form is completed, we should not immediately walk away. It is important to stand in the final stance awhile and feel the ch'i circulate.

Fig. A-105

Note

1. The starting direction is arbitrarily defined to be north.

Bibliography

Apel, Willi, *Harvard Dictionary of Music,* The Belknap Press of Harvard University Press, Cambridge, MA, 1969.

Bateson, F. W., *Selected Poems of William Blake,* Heinemann Press, London, 1978.

Chang, Jolan, *The Tao of Love and Sex,* E. P. Dutton, New York, NY, 1977.

Chang, Stephen T., Dr., *The Tao of Sexology,* Tao Publishing Co., San Francisco, CA, 1986.

Chen, William C. C., *Body Mechanics of T'ai Chi Ch'uan,* William C. C. Chen Publisher, New York, NY, 1973.

Chen, Yearning K., *Tai Chi Chuan—Its Effects and Practical Applications,* Ohara Publications, Los Angeles, CA, (no date).

Cheng Man-ch'ing and Robert Smith, *T'ai Chi,* Charles E. Tuttle Co., Rutland VT, 1967.

Cheng Man-ch'ing, *Cheng Tzu's Thirteen Treatises on Tai Chi Chuan,* Translated by Benjamin Pang-Jenny Lo and Martin Inn, North Atlantic Books, Berkeley, CA, 1985

Cheng Man-ch'ing, *T'ai Chi Ch'uan: A Simplified Method of Calisthenics & Self Defense,* North Atlantic Books, Berkeley, CA, 1981.

"Chi Disease! How You Can Get it, How You Can Prevent it!" *Inside Kung Fu,* Vol. 19, No. 10, October, 1992.

De Vries, Arnold, *Therapeutic Fasting,* Chandler Book Co., Los Angeles, CA, 1963.

Dement, William C., *Some Must Watch While Some Must Sleep,* W. W. Norton & Co., New York, NY, 1976.

"Dit Da Jow: Making Kung-Fu's Liquid Gold," *Inside Kung Fu,* Vol. 19, No. 10, October, 1992.

Dreisbach, Robert H., *Handbook of Poisoning,* Lange Medical Publications, Los Altos, CA, 1969.

Frantzis, Bruce Kumar, *Opening the Energy Gates of Your Body,* North Atlantic Books, Berkeley, CA, 1993.

Galante, Lawrence, *Tai Chi—The Supreme Ultimate,* Samuel Weiser, York Beach, ME, 1981.

Lao Tzu: "My words are easy to understand," *Lectures on the Tao Teh Ching by Man-Jan Cheng,* Translated by Tam C. Gibbs, North Atlantic Books, 1981.

LeBoyer, Frederick, *Birth Without Violence,* Alfred A. Knopf, New York, 1980.

"Liquid Gold or Fool's Potion?" *Inside Kung Fu,* Vol. 19, No. 7, July, 1992.

Pascal, Blaise, *Lettres Provinciales,* 14 Dec, 1656.

Ramacharaka, Yogi, *Science of Breath,* Yogi Publication Society, Chicago, IL. 1904, (ISBN 0-911662-00-6), available from Wheman Bros. Hackensack, NJ.

Roget, Peter Mark, *Roget's International Thesaurus,* HarperCollins Publishers, New York, NY, 1992.

Satchidananda, Yogiraj Sri Swami, *Integral Yoga Hatha,* Holt, Rinehart, and Winston, New York, 1970.

Scholem, Gershom, *Kabbalah,* Keter Publishing House, Jerusalem, 1974.

Shelton, Herbert M., *Food Combining Made Easy,* Dr. Shelton's Health School, San Antonio, TX, 1972.

Smith, Robert W., *Chinese Boxing: Masters and Methods,* Kodansha International, Ltd., Tokyo, 1974.

Smith, Robert W., *Pa-Kua: Chinese Boxing for Fitness and Self-defense,* Kodansha International Ltd., Tokyo, Japan, 1967.

T'ai Chi Ch'uan, Body and Mind, published by the T'ai Chi Ch'uan Association to commemorate its third anniversary in 1968.

The Essence of T'ai Chi Ch'uan: The Literary Tradition, Edited by Benjamin Pang-Jeng Lo et al., North Atlantic Books, Berkeley, CA, 1985.

Todd, M.D., Gary Price, *Nutrition,* Health, & Disease, Whitford Press, West Chester, PA, 1985.

Tseng Chiu-Yien, *The Chart of Tai Chi Chuan,* Union Press Limited, 14, Dorset Crescent, Kowloon Tong, Kowloon, Hong Kong.

United States Department of Agriculture, *Composition of Foods,* U. S. Government Printing Office, Washington, DC, 1963.

White, George M., *Craft Manual of North American Indian Footwear,* available from George M. White, P.O. Box 365, Ronan, Montana 59864.

Yang Jwing-Ming, *Muscle/Tendon Changing and Marrow/Brain Washing Chi Kung—The Secret of Youth,* Yang's Martial Arts Association, Jamaica Plain, MA, 1989.

Yang Zhen-Duo, *Traditional Yang Family Style Taijiquan,* A Taste of China, Inc., 111 Shirley Street, Winchester, VA 22601, 1991.

Index

Action and reaction, see Newton's third law
Acupuncture, 18, 20
Aerobic exercise, 148
Ahn, Don, 69
Air, 28
Alignment; *see also* Centering
and shearing stress, 66, 72, 89
cautions about, 89-90
importance of, 7
necessity of studying, 66-67
obstacles to reversing faulty patterns, 68
of ankle, 72
of arch of foot, 72
of elbows, 73
of hand, 70
of head, 73
of knees, 70-72
of pelvis, 73
of shoulders, 73
of spine, 73-74
of wrist, 70
parallel feet, 72-73
story about an acquaintance, 69
story, personal, 68-69
Ankle, see Alignment
Arch of foot; *see also* Alignment, 72
Arches, fallen
effect of excessive weight on, 133
harm caused by, 131-132
rehabilitation of, 132
Art and T'ai Chi Ch'uan, 141-144
Attitude, see Push-hands
Attentiveness, 8-9, 11, 52, 158
Axis of a bone, definition of, 70-71, 85
Balance; *see also* Equilibrium, Stability
and inner stability, 9

exercises for improving, 103-104
how we sense imbalance, 30-31
of opponent, 165-166
of left and right sides, 31-32
Beauteous hand, 33, 70; *see also* Alignment of Hand
Becque, Don Oscar, 33, 75
Being in the moment, 8-9, 11-12, 36
Blake, William, 45
Books learning from, 119-120
Breathing
abdominal, 59-61
and childbirth, 59-60
and the absorption of oxygen to the brain, 60-61
the importance of efficient, 58-59
exercise, 61-62
in T'ai Chi Ch'uan, 62-65
inefficient, the reasons for, 59-60
natural pattern of, 63
patterns, different, a reconciliation of, 63-65
Center line of foot, 83
Centering, 12, 30, 32-33, 70, 85, 102
Center of mass, 29-30; and alignment, 70
Chakras, 59
Ch'i; *see also* Ch'i Kung
and fixations of muscles, 4
and stretching, 76
benefits of, 19, 76-77
cautions about, 24-25
disruption and reinstatement of, 19
effect of clothing on, 23
experiencing, 19-20
failure to experience, 21
from inanimate objects, 23-24
in meditation, 4

scientific basis of, 20-21
sending of, 22-23
sensing and cultivating, 21-22
Ch'i kung, 18-19, 25, 85, 139, 189
Chen, William, C. C., xi, xiv, 27, 62, 91, 98, 156, 170, 173
Cheng Man-ch'ing, ii, xi, 1, 9, 13, 15, 18, 27, 54, 62-63, 70, 74, 85-86, 91-92, 95, 98, 102, 110, 118, 122, 128, 145-147, 150, 152, 157, 166-167, 172, 176-203
Childbirth, see Breathing
Chin Na, 38, 66-67, 169
Circles, 33-34, 102, 163
Classics, T'ai Chi Ch'uan, 11-14, 25, 35, 40, 44
Clothing
effect on breathing, 59
effect on Ch'i, 23
Compression of the form, 49, 98-99
Concentration, 11-13, 34-35, 95-96, 100
Continuity of practice, 92-93
Cool-down of leg muscles, 107
Coordination, 6-7, 9, 91, 102, 120
Dance and T'ai Chi Ch'uan, 144
Death, 11
Dit da jow, 125
Double weighting, 36, 84-85
Drawing silk, 36
Dreams, 55, 120-121
Eating before or after practice, 94, 106-107
Einstein, Albert, 46
Elbows, alignment of, 73
Endurance, 6
Energy, mechanical
conservation of, 42-43

converting translational into rotational, 43-44
kinetic, 43
potential, 43
Equilibrium
in push-hands, 29, 163-164
stable, neutral, and unstable, 29-30, 163, 167
Extensibility, 6
Fa Chin, 158
Feet; *see also* Arches, Stances, 36, 51, 72-73, 83-88, 103-104, 129-135, 138, 150-151
exercises of, 133
Feldenkreis, Moshe, 67-68
Feng Shui, 24
Flexibility
arresting or reversing loss of, 79
importance of, 75-78
reason for loss of, 75
Folding, see Push-hands, 160-161
Footwear, 67, 130-134
Force; *see also* Newton's third law, Push-hands
correct, 152, 154-155
use of too much, 164
Fountain, Marilyn, 7, 23
Galante, Lawrence, 9
Galileo's principle (Newton's first law), 38-39
Gate, 73, 169, 191
Ginseng, 137
Goal orientation, 5-6, 113-115, 172
Grabbing, 169-170
Gravity, 29-31, 37, 39
Grossman, Neal, 41
Hand, see Alignment
Head, alignment of, 73
Head, suspension of, 53-54
Healing, 5-9
Holtman, Alice, 22-23, 118
Images, 118
Injuries
Ch'i, use of in treating, 125
cold, application of, 125
cuts, 8, 125, 127

broken bones, 7, 125-126
bruises, 7, 19, 126
infections, 127
massage, use of in treating, 8, 127-129
rubs, 128-129
scrapes, 127
sprains, 7, 19, 74, 126
tendonitis, 126-127
treatment of, 123-129
Investment in loss, 14, 172-173
Joints; *see also* Alignment
cracking of, 82
thigh, 85-86, 40-41, 148
Journal, keeping a, 121
Karate, 15, 63, 147
Ki, see Ch'i
Kiai, 64-65
Kleinsmith, Lou, 173
Knee; *see also* Alignment, Stances
alignment of, 70-72
alignment of in 100% stance, 89
buckling of, 41, 89, 102
cautions about caving in of, 89
maximum extension of in stance, 87
Krishnamurti, J., 4
Kung Fu, 6,
Lao Tzu (quotes from Tao Te ch'ing)
Ch. 5, 25
Ch. 15, 16
Ch. 47, 15
Ch. 63, 11, 13
Ch. 78, 11
Learning process, the, 55, 95, 110-111, 113-121
LeBoyer, Charles, 60
Levelness of motion, 37-38
Leverage, 38
Liang, T. T., 110
Listening, see Push-hands
Lo, Benjamin, 110
Long form, 143, 145-146
Loss, investment in, see Investment in loss, 14, 172-173

Macrosco[...] mover[...]
Massage; [...] 67, 7[...]
Meditati[...] 24, [...]
Memor[...]
Meridi[...]
Metronome, practice, 105
Microsleep, 138-139
Mirror image of form, practice of, 97-98
Mirror, use of during practice, 104-105
Music; use of during practice, 105
Names of postures, 143, 177
Naps, 137-138
Neutralization, 15, 150, 152-154, 162-169, 171
minimum force in, 154-158
before returning, 156-157, 162
Newton's first law, 38-39
Newton's third law, 39-40, 155, 164-165
Non-action
principle of, 12-13, 148
in push-hands, 159-160
in self-defense, 13
Non-intention
principle of, 14, 159-160
in vision, 54-55
Notes, taking in class, 121
Nutrition, 123, 135
Opposite palms, see Push-hands, 161, 168
Pa-Kua Chang, 109
Pain, 124
Palming, 130
Pascal, Blaise, 12
Patience, 3, 9, 91, 114-118
Pelvis, alignment of, 73
P'eng, 41, 151
Perfect masters, 112-113
Perfectionism, 116-117
Perpetual motion, 41-44
Perret, Madeleine, 5
Pillows, 139

s of body, definitions of,
83
Pliability, 6
Postures, descriptions of, 177-
203
Postures, names of, 143, 177
Postures, photographs of, 178-
203
Practice
    blindfolded, 98
    continuity of, 92-93
    duration of, 93-94
    eating before or after, 94,
    106-107
    group or individual, 93
    importance of, 91
    in everyday life, 105-106
    mental, 100
    mirror, use of a, 104-105
    metronome, use of a, 105
    music, use of, 105
    outdoors, 94, 99-100
    place of, 94, 99-100
    quasi static, 96-97
    speed of, 96-97
    time of day of, 94
Prana, see Ch'i, 18, 59
Precision, 12, 44
Pulling, see Push-hands, 159,
169
Punches, taking, 171-172
Push-hands, 150-175
    action and reaction in, 164-
    165
    attitude, 172-174
    circles, 163
    contacting an opponent in,
    151, 161-162
    controlling the opponent's
    balance in, 165-166
    cooperation, 172, 174
    correct force in; see also
    minimum force in, 152,
    154-155
    equilibrium in, 163-164
    feeding the beginner in,
    173-174
    folding, 160-161
    grabbing, 169-170
    investment in loss in, 172-
    173

    listening, 158-159
    minimum force in, use of,
    157-158
    moving, 152
    neutralization, 150, 152-
    154, 156, 158, 162-163,
    166-169, 171
    non-action in, 159-160
    one-handed, 150-151
    opposite palms in, 161
    pulling, 159, 168-169
    receiving energy in, 157
    replacement in, 160
    returning, 156-157, 162
    rooting and redirecting in,
    155-156
    speed in, use of, 170
    stance, 162-163
    stepping, 150, 168-170
    sticking, 158
    T'i fang, 166-168
    two-handed, 151-152
    uprooting, 160, 164-165
    yielding, 152-153
    yin and yang (concept of
    T'ai Chi) in, 152
Reaction, see Newton's third
law, 39-40, 164-165
Reflexes, 6-7, 91
Reincarnation, 11
Replacement, see Push-hands
Returning, see Push-hands
River, the long, 41
Rooting, exercises for, 102-103
Rooting and redirecting, see
Push-hands, 155-156
Rubs, 128-129
San Shou (two-person form),
32, 99
Sayad, Khaleel, 172
Science and T'ai Chi Ch'uan,
145
Self-defense, 14-15
Semicircular canals in ears (and
balance), 98
Sensitivity
    effect of the mind on, 45-
    46
Sequence of motion, 47-48
Sexuality, 135-137
Shadow movements, 85

Shape, 48
Shaw, George Bernard, 13
Shearing stress, see Alignment,
66, 72, 89
Shoulders, alignment of, 73
Sitting, proper, 74
Sleep
    amounts, 139
    naps, 137-138
Smith, Robert, 33, 57, 147
Sober, Harvey I., 32, 56, 63,
98, 109-110, 124, 148,
156
Spatial relations, 48-49
Speed, use of, see Push-hands,
170
Spine, alignment of, 73-74
Spirituality, 2-3
Stability; see also Balance,
Equilibrium
    mental, 9, 22, 31
    of inanimate objects, 29-30
    of people, 30-31
Stances, 83-90
    cautions about alignment
    of knee in, 85, 89-90
    definitions of terms, 83-84
    fifty-fifty, 85-86, 103
    and double weighting, 36,
    84-85
    meditative, 85-86
    with bent knees, 86
    with straight knees, 85
    in push-hands, see Push-
    hands, 162-163
    one-hundred-percent, 89
    seventy-thirty, 86-89
    knee, maximum extension
    of, 87-88
    seventy-thirty, diagonal,
    88-89
Stepping, 49-51
Stepping in, see Push-hands,
168-170
Sticking; see also Push-hands,
151, 158
Strength, 5-6, 52
Stretching, 76-81
    analogy to consensus at a
    meeting, 78
    benefits of, 76-79

best time of day for, 80
correct, importance of, 77-78
equally in both directions, 81
experiencing the effects of, 79
getting up after, 79-80
hanging, 81
monitoring progress of, 78
repeating, the importance of, 81
spontaneously, 80
using gravity, 80-81
using momentum, 81
Summers, Elaine, 20, 66, 68-69, 75, 110, 124, 127, 129, 132
Sung; in push-hands, 154-157, 172
Suspension of the head, 53-54
Swimming in air, 28
Taking punches, 171-172
Tan t'ien; see also Sung, 30, 53, 64
Teachers, 107-113
    asking questions of, 111
    attitude toward, 111-112
    choosing one, 107-108
    methods of, 108-111
Thigh joints, opening and closing of, 40-41
T'i fang, see Push-hands, 166-168
Timing, 9, 93, 95, 105, 120, 150, 155, 167
Taoism, 2-3, 10-15
Two-person form, see San Shou, 32, 99
Unity of movement, 50, 54
Uproot, see Push-hands, 36, 104, 156-157, 162, 164-166, 168, 170, 172-173
Valenti, Fernando, 146
Verticality of the axis of the body, 54
Videotape, learning from a, 119-120
Vision, 30-31, 130; and balance, 30-31

Visualization; in daily-life situations, 56-57
Wang Tsung-Yueh, 28, 40, 45
Warm-Up, 75-76, 78, 80, 82
Watson, Patrick, 156
Weber's law, 46, 157, 159
Weight distribution
    on foot, 30, 130-131
    in stances, 83-86
Words and speech, 117-118
Wrist, see Alignment, 70
Wu Yu-Hsiang, 49, 160
Yang Cheng-fu, 15, 63, 97, 145-146
Yang Lu-chan, 14-15
Yang Zhen-Duo, 63, 65, 205
Yawning, 80
Yielding, 3, 10-11, 41, 47, 64, 152-156, 159
Yin and yang
    general concept of, 10-12
    in push-hands, 150
    separation of, 46-47, 96, 103
Zen, 14

BOOKS & VIDEOS FROM YMAA

YMAA Publication Center Books

B041/868	101 Reflections on Tai Chi Chuan
B031/582	108 Insights into Tai Chi Chuan—A String of Pearls
B046/906	6 Healing Movements—Qigong for Health, Strength, & Longevity
B045/833	A Woman's Qigong Guide—Empowerment through Movement, Diet, and Herbs
B009/041	Analysis of Shaolin Chin Na—Instructor's Manual for all Martial Styles
B004R/671	Ancient Chinese Weapons—A Martial Artist's Guide
B015R/426	Arthritis—The Chinese Way of Healing and Prevention (formerly Qigong for Arthritis)
B030/515	Back Pain—Chinese Qigong for Healing and Prevention
B020/300	Baguazhang—Emei Baguazhang
B043/922	Cardio Kickboxing Elite—For Sport, for Fitness, for Self-Defense
B028/493	Chinese Fast Wrestling for Fighting—The Art of San Shou Kuai Jiao
B016/254	Chinese Qigong Massage—General Massage
B038/809	Complete CardioKickboxing—A Safe & Effective Approach to High Performance Living
B021/36x	Comprehensive Applications of Shaolin Chin Na—The Practical Defense of Chinese Seizing Arts for All Styles
B010R/523	Eight Simple Qigong Exercises for Health—The Eight Pieces of Brocade
B025/353	The Essence of Shaolin White Crane—Martial Power and Qigong
B014R/639	The Essence of Taiji Qigong—The Internal Foundation of Taijiquan (formerly Tai Chi Chi Kung)
B017R/345	How to Defend Yourself—Effective & Practical Martial Arts Strategies
B013/084	Hsing Yi Chuan—Theory and Applications
B033/655	The Martial Arts Athlete—Mental and Physical Conditioning for Peak Performance
B042/876	Mind/Body Fitness
B006R/85x	Northern Shaolin Sword—Forms, Techniques, and Applications
B044/914	Okinawa's Complete Karate System—Isshin-Ryu
B037/760	Power Body—Injury Prevention, Rehabilitation, and Sports Performance Enhancement
B050/99x	Principles of Traditional Chinese Medicine—The Essential Guide to Understanding the Human Body
B012R/841	Qigong—The Secret of Youth
B005R/574	Qigong for Health and Martial Arts—Exercises and Meditation (formerly Chi Kung—Health & Martial Arts)
B040/701	Qigong for Treating Common Ailments—The Essential Guide to Self-Healing
B011R/507	The Root of Chinese Qigong—Secrets for Health, Longevity, & Enlightenment
B049/930	Taekwondo—Ancient Wisdom for the Modern Warrior
B032/647	The Tai Chi Book—Refining and Enjoying a Lifetime of Practice
B019R/337	Tai Chi Chuan—24 & 48 Postures with Martial Applications (formerly Simplified Tai Chi Chuan)
B008R/442	Tai Chi Chuan Martial Applications—Advanced Yang Style (formerly Advanced Yang Style Tai Chi Chuan, v.2)
B035/71x	Tai Chi Secrets of the Ancient Masters—Selected Readings with Commentary
B047/981	Tai Chi Secrets of the Wŭ & Li Styles—Chinese Classics, Translations, Commentary
B048/094	Tai Chi Secrets of the Yang Style—Chinese Classics, Translations, Commentary
B007R/434	Tai Chi Theory & Martial Power—Advanced Yang Style (formerly Advanced Yang Style Tai Chi Chuan, v.1)
B022/378	Taiji Chin Na—The Seizing Art of Taijiquan
B036/744	Taiji Sword, Classical Yang Style—The Complete Form, Qigong, and Applications
B034/68x	Taijiquan, Classical Yang Style—The Complete Form and Qigong
B046/892	Traditional Chinese Health Secrets—The Essential Guide to Harmonious Living
B039/787	Wild Goose Qigong—Natural Movement for Healthy Living
B027/361	Wisdom's Way—101 Tales of Chinese Wit

YMAA Publication Center Videotapes

T004/211	Analysis of Shaolin Chin Na
T007/246	Arthritis—The Chinese Way of Healing and Prevention
T028/566	Back Pain—Chinese Qigong for Healing & Prevention
T033/086	Chin Na In Depth—Course One
T034/019	Chin Na In Depth—Course Two
T008/327	Chinese Qigong Massage—Self Massage
T009/335	Chinese Qigong Massage—With a Partner
T012/386	Comprehensive Applications of Shaolin Chin Na 1
T013/394	Comprehensive Applications of Shaolin Chin Na 2
T005/22x	Eight Simple Qigong Exercises for Health—The Eight Pieces of Brocade
T017/280	Emei Baguazhang 1—Basic Training, Qigong, Eight Palms, & Their Applications
T018/299	Emei Baguazhang 2—Swimming Body & Its Applications
T019/302	Emei Baguazhang 3—Bagua Deer Hook Sword & Its Applications
T006/238	The Essence of Taiji Qigong—The Internal Foundation of Taijiquan
T010/343	How to Defend Yourself 1—Unarmed Attack
T011/351	How to Defend Yourself 2—Knife Attack
T035/051	Northern Shaolin Sword—San Cai Jian and Its Applications
T036/06x	Northern Shaolin Sword—Kun Wu Jian and Its Applications
T037/078	Northern Shaolin Sword—Qi Men Jian and Its Applications
T029/590	The Scientific Foundation of Chinese Qigong—A Lecture by Dr. Yang, Jwing-Ming
T003/203	Shaolin Long Fist Kung Fu—Gung Li Chuan and Its Applications
T002/19x	Shaolin Long Fist Kung Fu—Lien Bu Chuan and Its Applications
T015/264	Shaolin Long Fist Kung Fu—Shi Zi Tang and Its Applications
T025/604	Shaolin Long Fist Kung Fu—Xiao Hu Yuan (Roaring Tiger Fist) and Its Applications
T014/256	Shaolin Long Fist Kung Fu—Yi Lu Mai Fu & Er Lu Mai Fu and Their Applications
T021/329	Simplified Tai Chi Chuan—Simplified 24 Postures & Standard 48 Postures
T022/469	Sun Style Taijiquan—With Applications
T024/485	Tai Chi Chuan & Applications—Simplified 24 Postures with Applications & Standard 48 Postures
T016/408	Taiji Chin Na
T031/817	Taiji Sword, Classical Yang Style—The Complete Form, Qigong, and Applications
T030/752	Taijiquan, Classical Yang Style—The Complete Form and Qigong
T026/612	White Crane Hard Qigong—The Essence of Shaolin White Crane
T027/620	White Crane Soft Qigong—The Essence of Shaolin White Crane
T032/949	Wild Goose Qigong—Natural Movement for Healthy Living
T023/477	Wu Style Taijiquan—With Applications
T020/310	Xingyiquan—The Twelve Animal Patterns & Their Applications
T001/181	Yang Style Tai Chi Chuan—and Its Applications

YMAA PUBLICATION CENTER 楊氏東方文化出版中心

4354 Washington Street Roslindale, MA 02131

1-800-669-8892 • ymaa@aol.com • www.ymaa.com